Pigmentation Disorders - Diagnosis and Management

Edited by Pierre Vereecken

Published in London, United Kingdom

Pigmentation Disorders - Diagnosis and Management
http://dx.doi.org/10.5772/intechopen.1008601
Edited by Pierre Vereecken

Contributors
Alfredo Martínez-Gutiérrez, Ana Maria Dascalu, Bingyu Wang, Bogdan-Stefan Negreanu-Pirjol, Florentina Nicoleta Roncea, Julia Aullo, Liyuan Zhou, Maria-Andrada Hincu, Maria Glushkova, Mari Carmen González, Marina Adriana Mercioni, Mihaela Cezarina Mehedinti, Mokgadi Ursula Makgobole, Neus Calbet-Llopart, Nina Ivanovic, Nomakhosi Mpofana, Olivia Toma, Pavitra Pillay, Peiru Wang, Qingyu Zeng, Raluca Dumache, Sanda Jurja, Shuzhan Shen, Ticuta Negreanu-Pirjol, Xidie Yin, Xiuli Wang, Yiting Zhao, Zhi Cao

First published in London, United Kingdom, 2026 by IntechOpen
IntechOpen is the global imprint of INTECHOPEN LIMITED, registered in England and Wales, registration number: 11086078, 167-169 Great Portland Street, London, W1W 5PF, United Kingdom

For EU product safety concerns: IN TECH d.o.o., Prolaz Marije Krucifikse Kozulić 3, 51000 Rijeka, Croatia, info@intechopen.com or visit our website at intechopen.com.

British Library Cataloguing-in-Publication Data
A catalogue record for this book is available from the British Library

Pigmentation Disorders - Diagnosis and Management
Edited by Pierre Vereecken
p. cm.
Print ISBN 978-1-83635-692-9
Online ISBN 978-1-83635-691-2
eBook (PDF) ISBN 978-1-83635-693-6

Meet the editor

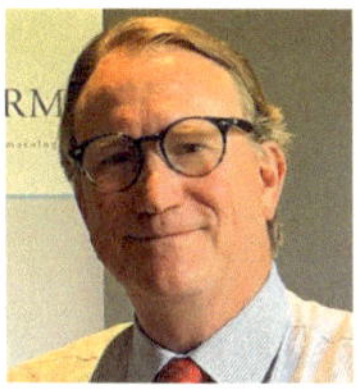

Dr. Pierre Vereecken, MD, Ph.D., is qualified and specialized in Dermatology (general, aesthetic, and corrective) and in cutaneous oncology. He studied medicine at the University of Brussels, Belgium (1991), and obtained his Ph.D. from the same university in 2008, with research on cutaneous malignant melanoma biology and progression. In 2010, Dr. Pierre Vereecken founded Cliderm (Clinics in Dermatology), an international network of dermatologists, and the European Institute for Dermatology Practice and Research. This multifaceted organization aims to promote clinical dermatology and dermatology research worldwide. He has published more than 100 scientific papers in international medical literature and also edited and authored chapters for more than 20 books.

Contents

Preface

Pigmentary disorders are various skin conditions that affect the color of the skin. They can result from various causes, including genetic factors, sun exposure, autoimmune diseases, or hormonal imbalances. The most common disorders include vitiligo, characterized by white patches on the skin due to the destruction of melanocytes, the cells that produce melanin. Other pigmentary disorders include melasma, a well-known facial pigmentation disorder, lentigines, brown spots caused by excessive sun exposure, and melanomas, an aggressive form of skin cancer that can appear as abnormal moles. Individuals with pigmentary disorders may experience aesthetic and psychological concerns due to the appearance of their skin.

The treatment for pigmentary disorders varies depending on the specific condition. Options such as lightening creams, laser therapies, or even skin grafts may be considered. It is essential to consult a dermatologist for an appropriate diagnosis and tailored treatment plan. Adequate sun protection is also crucial to prevent the worsening of pigmentary disorders.

In this book, we gathered important and varied aspects of pigmentation disorders, and we hope to offer new perspectives in the near future, thanks to the experts who agreed to collaborate on this project.

Pierre Vereecken
Cliderm Clinics Dermatology,
Brussels, Belgium

Chapter 1

A Multifaceted and Holistic Protocol for the Treatment of Skin Hyperpigmentation: Targeting Melanin Removal, Inhibition, and Cellular Signaling

Alfredo Martínez-Gutiérrez, Neus Calbet-Llopart, Julia Aullo and Mari Carmen González

Abstract

Hyperpigmentation is a multifactorial dermatological condition requiring a comprehensive and layered treatment approach that addresses various physiological aspects of the skin. Effective management demands targeting not only visible pigmentation but also the underlying mechanisms driving its development and persistence. Recognizing that hyperpigmentation arises from both intrinsic and extrinsic influences – including inflammation, hormonal triggers, and ultraviolet (UV) exposure – therapeutic strategies must consider epidermal turnover, melanogenesis, cellular signaling, and the aging microenvironment. Here, we describe the key steps for skin hyperpigmentation regulation (removal of existing melanin, melanogenesis regulation in the melanocyte, regulation of paracrine melanogenic factors, photoprotection, and oral supplements) and propose a multifaceted and holistic protocol that integrates these different steps for the successful management of skin hyperpigmentation conditions.

Keywords: hyperpigmentation, melanin, tyrosinase, cellular signaling, paracrine regulation, translational approach

1. Introduction

Skin pigmentation is mainly affected by the amount of melanin pigment present in the epidermis, the upper layer of the skin. In the basal layer of the epidermis, we find melanocytes, a dendritic cell with the ability to synthesize melanin from the amino acid L-tyrosine in specialized organelles called melanosomes. Here, the rate-limiting enzyme tyrosinase (TYR) participates in several steps of the melanin production process. First, TYR catalyzes the formation of L-DOPA from L-tyrosine and then the formation of dopaquinone from L-DOPA, with this last one being the rate-limiting step [1].

After this point, the production of melanin can take two directions, which depend on the presence of cysteine. When cysteine is absent, eumelanin forms, which is a high molecular weight form of quinones derived from dopaquinone that polymerize together to form the dark brown-black pigment, possessing high photoprotection capabilities. Instead, if cysteine is present, the polymerization of intermediates results in the formation of pheomelanin, a red to yellow pigment that is less photoprotective and can promote reactive oxygen species (ROS) formation under ultraviolet (UV) exposure. The ratio of these types of melanin determines the skin tone and consequently the intrinsic ability of skin to protect against UV damage [2].

Once melanin is formed, melanosomes are transferred from melanocytes to keratinocytes through an intricate network of microtubule and actin-mediated transport proteins. Once melanosomes are endocytosed by keratinocytes, these organelles localize upon the cell nucleus, forming a cap-like structure and acting as a photoprotective "umbrella" against UV-induced damage in the nuclear DNA [3].

As detailed in this chapter, both melanin synthesis and distribution are dynamically regulated by genetic, hormonal, and environmental factors. These factors primarily act by inducing ROS levels in skin cells, which upregulate a wide range of cytokines and proinflammatory genes. Afterward, these paracrine proteins released by keratinocytes (α-MSH, endothelin-1, PGE2) or fibroblasts (SCF, HGF) can bind to different receptors on melanocytes, consequently activating intracellular pathways such as PKA, MAPK/ERK, or PI3K/Akt [4]. Interestingly, all these pathways converge in the upregulation and activation of microphthalmia-associated transcription factor (MITF), a transcription factor that controls the gene expression of the key enzymes involved in melanogenesis [5].

Interestingly, all these pathways are shared in the different hyperpigmentation conditions. However, what makes the difference in each condition is the specific contribution or key role in the pathophysiology of each pathway. **Table 1** summarizes the key pathways involved in the most common hyperpigmentation conditions:

Given this complex regulation of melanogenesis through this intricate network of proteins and pathways, hyperpigmentation management needs to be approached through combinatorial strategies that target multiple pathways. The next sections describe in detail how each of these steps is key for hyperpigmentation and how they can be regulated using specific strategies or compounds:

Type	Key pathophysiological drivers	References
Melasma	Hormonal fluctuations (estrogen/progesterone), UV exposure, vascular hyperactivity (VEGF), and oxidative stress.	[6, 7]
Post-inflammatory hyper-pigmentation (PIH)	Inflammatory cytokines (IL-1α, IL-6, TNF-α), prostaglandins, and leukotrienes result from skin trauma or dermatitis.	[8, 9]
Solar lentigines	Chronic UV-induced DNA damage and senescence-associated secretory phenotype (SASP) in keratinocytes.	[10]

Table 1.
Types of skin hyperpigmentation conditions and key pathophysiological drivers involved in each process.

- Elimination of existing melanin deposits through peelings, retinol, and autophagy activators
- Melanogenesis inhibition within the melanocyte occurs through TYR inhibition and other melanocyte-specific pathways
- Regulation of paracrine factors from neighboring cells that stimulate melanocytes
- Photoprotection and topical antioxidant use to prevent promelanogenic and proinflammatory pathway activation.
- Oral whitening, antioxidant, and photoprotective compounds.

In the following sections, each phase of this multi-pronged therapeutic strategy will be detailed, with emphasis on mechanisms of action, active ingredients, clinical evidence, and practical application protocols.

2. Elimination of existing melanin deposits in the epidermis

In certain pigmentary disorders, such as solar lentigines and age spots, melanin is predominantly accumulated in the upper epidermal layers, especially within keratinocytes. This is distinct from melasma, where melanocytes themselves tend to be the primary site of hyperactivity and melanosome accumulation [11, 12]. The therapeutic approach in these cases should prioritize enhanced epidermal turnover and stratum corneum exfoliation to eliminate excess pigment. Several options are available to manage this level of pigmentation regulation:

Chemical peelings: These types of topical solutions are based on the use of acid compounds that interact with the epidermal keratinocyte intercellular connections, which favor cellular shedding and consequently epidermal exfoliation [13]. Thus, the chemically induced epidermal remodeling produces not only the elimination of melanin granules but also a significant improvement in skin quality. Depending on the type of acid and concentration, chemical peels can be classified as superficial, medium, or deep. Medium and deep peels are designed to reach the dermis and produce significant skin remodeling changes, including addressing conditions such as photoaging or scars, among others [14]. Regarding epidermal hyperpigmentation, superficial peels are commonly the chosen ones to induce epidermal desquamation. For superficial peels, the typical acids to be used are detailed in **Table 2**. Common final formulations include a combination of these acids and other ingredients to significantly boost clinical efficacy [15].

Interestingly, tranexamic acid is another acid included in peeling formulations to boost the depigmenting effect [16]. Although it is not an exfoliating acid per se, its multimodal mechanism of action in skin pigmentation regulation (mainly vascularization and inflammation control) has led to its administration via different routes, as will be described in the next sections, including oral, injected, and microneedling applications.

Retinoids: The retinoid family includes a wide range of vitamin A derivatives that regulate many skin processes through their binding to the retinoic acid receptor (RAR) family [24]. Among these, RAR activation promotes epidermal turnover by

Acid	Concentration in chemical peelings	References
Salicylic acid	20%–30%	[17, 18]
Glycolic acid	30%–70%	[19–21]
Trichloroacetic acid	10%–20%	[22]
Kojic acid	Up to 10%	[23]

Table 2.
Main acids and their concentrations used in chemical peelingpeelings formulations to promote epidermal exfoliation and renewal in skin hyperpigmentation conditions.

accelerating epidermal proliferation and differentiation steps at the different sublayers of the epidermis. Consequently, the epidermal layer is thickened, and renewal is accelerated [25]. This process is known as "retinization" and is a key factor to consider when using retinoids on the skin, as it can be followed by mild adverse effects in some cases. Thus, the increase in keratinocyte shedding induced by this promoted epidermal renewal contributes to melanin granule elimination in the upper layers of the skin. Several studies have proven the efficacy of using retinoids to accelerate melanin elimination, both as a single therapy and as part of a combination protocol with other topical products [26]. A practical tip when starting the use of retinoids on the skin is applying the product on alternate nights during the first week of treatment and progressively increasing to daily applications to help the skin adapt to the accelerated epidermal turnover and minimize irritation and barrier disruption. As for the available vitamin A derivatives, retinol, retinol esters, retinal, or hydroxypinacolone retinoate are among the most used in over-the-counter formulations based on their efficacy and tolerability profile [27].

Autophagy activators: Autophagy is an intracellular degradation pathway essential for recycling cytoplasmic components and maintaining cellular homeostasis [28]. Impaired autophagy contributes to pigment accumulation and cellular senescence in aged skin. In fact, previous studies have shown that autophagy activation can promote melanosome degradation, thus reducing the amount of existing melanin in both keratinocytes and melanocytes [29]. To date, several ingredients have been described as activators of autophagy in skin cells with the purpose of reducing melanin levels (see **Table 3**).

Compound	Effect on autophagy in epidermal cells	References
Trehalose	Autophagy induction in HaCaT keratinocytes	[30]
Ectoin	Autophagy induction in B16F10 melanocytes and HaCaT keratinocytes	[31]
3-o-ethyl ascorbic acid	Autophagy induction in B16F10 melanocytes	[32]
Coenzyme q0	Autophagy induction in HaCaT keratinocytes and zebrafish model	[33]
Pterostilbene	Autophagy induction in HaCaT keratinocytes	[34]
Apigenin + Phloretin	Upregulation of autophagy-related genes in human primary melanocytes	[35]

Table 3.
Compounds that can activate autophagy in epidermal cells, according to previous research.

Laser-based melanin elimination: Energy-based devices that use lasers, mainly Q-switched Nd:YAG lasers, are also commonly used to eliminate existing melanin deposits by causing photothermolysis of the melanosomes without damaging melanocytes. These lasers are usually combined with other topical treatments to boost efficacy and reduce adverse effects associated with laser use [36].

Despite the promising results of the above studies, many of the aforementioned compounds have not been tested in clinical studies, so clinical efficacy remains unknown.

In this context, a combination of the three strategies (chemical peeling, retinoids, and autophagy activators) in medically specialized protocols seems to be the best approach to work synergistically and optimize clinical outcomes. For example, several chemical peeling sessions, combined with a topical homecare routine including retinoids and autophagy activators between sessions, could be used to remove superficial melanin accumulations in solar lentigos or to prepare the skin for stronger topical or device-associated procedures aimed at regulating melasma pathology [37]. In fact, previous studies have shown promising results when combining, for example, peelings with topical regimens including retinoids and other ingredients [17, 38, 39].

3. Melanogenesis inhibition and control within the melanocyte

Once the existing deposits of melanin have been addressed, and in parallel to this first step, it is key to start modulating the hyperactivity of melanocytes. Hyperpigmentation conditions, such as melasma, are chronic conditions, which means that the treatment must address the constant activation of melanocytes by different stimuli [7]. Thus, inhibiting the production of melanin in the melanocyte is as important as eliminating the already existing melanin in the upper layers.

Melanogenesis is a complex, multi-step biological process that culminates in the production of melanin within melanocytes. The process is initiated by the enzymatic oxidation of the amino acid L-tyrosine into dopaquinone, catalyzed by the copper-dependent enzyme TYR. This step represents the rate-limiting phase of melanogenesis. Dopaquinone undergoes further transformations, ultimately resulting in the synthesis of eumelanin or pheomelanin, depending on the presence of cysteine and other cofactors [5].

TYR is transcriptionally regulated by the MITF, a master regulator in pigment cell development and function. MITF itself is controlled by several signaling cascades, including the MAPK, PI3K/Akt, and Wnt/β-catenin pathways. These pathways respond to external stimuli such as UV radiation and inflammatory cytokines, integrating environmental inputs with gene expression responses [4].

Consequently, we identified two proteins that are considered key in the production of melanin from the molecular point of view: MITF and TYR. Both proteins are melanocyte-specific and are located downstream of all the molecular pathways that can activate melanogenesis in the melanocyte.

TYR has historically been chosen as a common target for the testing and design of ingredients to inhibit melanogenesis [40]. Both natural and synthetic compounds show good efficacy at blocking TYR enzymatic activity, with a plethora of different mechanisms, including copper chelation at the active site, competitive enzymatic inhibition, non-competitive inhibitors, or mixed inhibitors [41]. Among the studies published on TYR inhibition, many used the well-known mushroom TYR, based on the fast, cheap, and easy availability of the enzyme to test whether a compound shows TYR inhibition properties. However, later studies showed that mushroom and human TYR have significant structural differences, meaning that extrapolation from mushroom TYR inhibition to human TYR inhibition should not be assumed to be straightforward [42].

Regarding MITF, its structural complexity as a transcriptional factor makes it challenging to be targeted by small molecules. Thus, a few molecules have been described to inhibit MITF [43]. Instead, compounds that block MITF gene expression have arisen alternatively as a specific mechanism of melanogenesis blockage.

In addition to transcriptional control, TYR activity is regulated at the post-translational level through glycosylation, phosphorylation, and intracellular trafficking. These modifications can both block proper enzymatic function or target the TYR protein for degradation. Thus, targeting TYR directly, or its upstream regulators, offers multiple avenues for therapeutic intervention in pigmentary conditions.

Other suggested pathways for melanogenesis regulation include epigenetic mechanisms. Among these, miRNAs play a key role in regulating the gene expression of key proteins such as MITF or TYR. Specifically, miRNAs are small RNAs (21–23 nucleotides in length) that bind to the messenger RNA of specific genes to block the corresponding expression of that gene, serving as a highly conserved mechanism to control pigmentation gene expression. Particularly, miR-203, miR-145, miR-137, miR-218, and miR-675 are among the miRNAs that target melanogenesis-specific genes such as MITF, TYR, TYRP1, or TYRP2.

Table 4 shows different compounds that regulate melanogenesis in the melanocyte according to the previously explained mechanisms of action. These compounds are among the commonly available options to be included in topical products aimed at blocking melanocyte function.

Of note, hydroquinone has been historically defined as a TYR inhibitor, thereby justifying its clinical efficacy. However, studies have shown that hydroquinone is a weak TYR inhibitor and rather acts by inducing melanocyte damage and necrosis, which translates into a significant depigmenting effect but is accompanied by severe adverse effects such as ochronosis or excessive hypopigmentation [53, 54]. This has prompted the search for alternative depigmenting compounds that effectively

Mechanism of melanogenesis regulation in the melanocyte	Compounds	References
Tyrosinase inhibitors	Hydroquinone*, Kojic acid, arbutin, epigallocatechin gallate, glabridin, resorcinols, azelaic acid, chalcone-derivatives, retinol	[41, 44, 45]
Tyrosinase post-translational modifications and/or increased degradation	4-n-butyl resorcinol, linoleic acid, resveratrol, n-acetyl glucosamine	[46–48]
MITF inhibitor/MITF downregulation	Lipoic acid, hesperidin, glabridin, resveratrol, polydeoxyribonucleotide (PDRN)	[49–52]
Epigenetic regulation	Apigenin, Chalcone-derivative	[35, 44]

Table 4.
List of compounds that block melanogenesis in the melanocyte, classified by mechanism of action.

lighten skin without incurring adverse effects, with those detailed in **Table 4** representing the most frequently employed options.

Besides the previously described melanogenesis regulatory mechanisms, melanosome transfer from melanocytes to keratinocytes has also been widely studied as a depigmenting mechanism. However, this mechanism alone does not exert a significant effect in reducing pigmentation in the skin and needs to be complemented with other mechanisms, such as the ones already explained. Regarding compounds acting on this pathway, niacinamide seems to be the gold standard for blocking melanosome transfer. Considering the efficacy of niacinamide as a skin-whitening agent, it is probable that this depigmenting efficacy is also based on its other mechanisms of action, including antioxidant and anti-inflammatory properties [55].

Finally, many of the previously mentioned compounds have multitarget mechanisms covering other important functions such as inflammation control, photoprotection, or antioxidation, as described in the next sections.

4. Regulation of paracrine factors that stimulate melanocytes

As previously mentioned, external damage, such as UV radiation, can trigger the production of proinflammatory cytokines, growth factors, and prostaglandins in skin cells such as keratinocytes and fibroblasts. These cytokines can act on neighboring melanocytes to stimulate and induce melanin production. This effect is known as the paracrine effect, and it is a key step for hyperpigmentation control.

After reviewing existing melanin deposits and melanogenesis inside the melanocyte, these paracrine factors released by damaged skin cells offer a new level of pigmentation control. Interestingly, this is also a feature shared by the different types of skin hyperpigmentation conditions. Solar lentigos, melasma, and post-inflammatory hyperpigmentation share the upregulated levels of proteins such as stem cell factor (SCF), endothelin-1 (ET-1), or α-melanocyte-stimulating hormone (α-MSH), among others [11, 56, 57].

Epidermal melanocytes possess membrane receptors for these cytokines, each of them triggering intracellular responses that result in increased activation of MITF, and consequently, increased production of melanogenesis-related enzymes. Thus, compounds that prevent the production of these proinflammatory factors and/or block their promelanogenic effect through their cellular receptors are another key tool in the skin hyperpigmentation management protocol. As expected, this will play a major role in the maintenance part of the protocol to prevent repigmentation.

The most used and better-known topical ingredients for the regulation of paracrine factors in the skin are detailed in **Table 5**.

Regarding other paracrine mechanisms involved in skin pigmentation, estrogens were long thought to stimulate melanocytes directly. However, recent data suggest that vascular changes (e.g., increased VEGF and endothelins) mediate most of the pigmentary effects seen in melasma [69, 70] Finally, recent studies highlight the role of sebocytes as contributors to the secretion of these promelanogenic paracrine factors [71]. Further research to test whether the currently used depigmenting compounds or novel compounds regulate sebocyte activity is warranted.

Ingredient/s	Paracrine regulation mechanism	References
Retinol + ferulic acid + diosmin	Reduction of promelanogenic ET-1 and COX-2, and stimulation of anti-melanogenic IL-1b in dermal fibroblasts	[58]
Astaxanthin	Reduction of interleukin-1α, interleukin-6/8, GM-CSF, and ET-1 in HaCaT keratinocytes Blockage of SCF-induced melanogenesis	[59, 60]
Chamomile extract	Blockage of ET-1-induced melanogenesis	[57]
Ashwagandha extract	Blockage of SCF and ET-1-induced melanogenesis	[61]
Tranexamic acid	Inhibition of plasminogen activation, reducing keratinocyte-derived melanogenic factors ET-1 downregulation in endothelial cells	[62, 63]
Hexylresorcinol	Inflammation downregulation through NF–kB inhibition	[64, 65]
Glabridin/licorice extract	Inflammation downregulation through cyclooxygenase and NF-κB inhibition Inhibition of Wnt pathway	[66, 67]
Niacinamide	Inflammation downregulation through NF–kB inhibition	[55]
Apigenin + Phloretin	Inhibition of Wnt-stimulated melanogenesis Upregulation of DKK1 (Wnt inhibitor) and downregulation of VEGF in dermal fibroblasts	[35]
Glucosamine	Inhibition of ET-1 + SCF-induced melanogenesis	[68]

Table 5.
List of compounds that regulate melanogenesis through the control of paracrine mechanisms as described in previous research

5. Topical photoprotection and antioxidant use

Protection against UV damage from sun exposure is the next level of hyperpigmentation control. Following the regulatory pathways previously described, we find ROS as the trigger for the proinflammatory cytokines that stimulate melanocytes [72]. Thus, photoprotection is key to preventing ROS production and consequently the downstream signaling. In fact, the shared features of melasma with photoaging reveal the importance of sun exposure and damage in these conditions [7].

Historically, photoprotection was limited to preventing UVA and UVB damage to the skin. However, research has shown that visible light (mainly solar blue light) plays a key role in both promoting skin aging and hyperpigmentation. Blue light possesses the ability to increase ROS levels and activate opsin-3 receptors in melanocytes, which, in turn, activates the melanogenic pathway. Considering the key role of ROS in the visible light-mediated promelanogenic effect, antioxidants offer a good complement to UVA/UVB filters for complete photoprotection against sun exposure. In conclusion, photoprotection for hyperpigmentation management must cover UVA, UVB, and visible light protection.

Besides the already known UVA/UVB filters, here we mention some antioxidants and visible-light blockers to be used in a full-coverage photoprotection approach:

- Tinted sunscreens (iron oxide, titanium oxide): these compounds provide a physical barrier by blocking visible light by 93%–98% [73]. There are already several clinical studies proving the prevention of visible light-induced pigmentation by using these sunscreens when exposed to sunlight [74, 75].

- Glutathione: topical glutathione at doses from 0.5% to 2% has shown clinical benefits on melasma skin [76]. The combination with microneedling and oral supplementation can boost the results of topical glutathione monotherapy.

- Vitamin C: topical vitamin C has been widely used not only to reduce signs of skin aging but also to enhance skin brightening and diminish the appearance of pigmentation spots. The highest effective dose, while maintaining a good safety profile, is around 15%, as higher doses (20% and more) do not provide greater efficacy and can even increase adverse effects, such as mild irritation [77]. Interestingly, vitamin C can also contribute to mitigating the damaging effects of blue light on the skin [78].

- Niacinamide: as in the case of vitamin C, niacinamide can contribute to the protection against blue light-induced damage [79].

- Idebenone: a synthetic analog of coenzyme Q10 with strong antioxidant properties, which also acts as a melanogenesis blocker in the melanocyte and has anti-inflammatory properties [80].

- Mycosporine-like amino acids (MAAs): these are compounds produced by many marine organisms with the ability to absorb UV light. These natural compounds are being increasingly incorporated into sunscreens based on their good safety profile and efficacy, boosting the photoprotection of current synthetic sunscreens [81].

Interestingly, these antioxidants are topically applied to the skin as part of creams, serums, or sprays. However, vehiculation of these ingredients in transepithelial solutions using microneedling and/or mesotherapy has also shown good clinical results [82]. Microneedling itself has been suggested to positively impact depigmenting results, meaning that a possible synergistic effect might occur by combining microneedling with topical antioxidants.

6. Oral whitening, photoprotectors, and antioxidants

The compounds mentioned in the previous sections show great results when applied topically to prevent and/or treat hyperpigmentation spots on the skin. Noteworthy, some of these compounds have also been studied for oral supplementation with different objectives, such as increasing depigmenting and/or photoprotection action at the systemic level. Thus, this is believed to boost the effect of topically applied compounds and act synergistically to reduce skin pigmentation. It is important to remark that, while oral photoprotection cannot substitute topical photoprotection, it offers a good complement to achieve successful protection of the skin against sun damage.

On the contrary, recent evidence on the relationship between melasma and oxidative stress supports this approach of combining oral and topical treatments. Previous studies have shown that systemic oxidative stress levels are increased, while endogenous antioxidant levels are decreased in melasma patients [83–85]. Oral photoprotectors are included in this section, as there is compelling evidence showing that they can boost skin protection against sunlight damage, as demonstrated in clinical studies [86]. Here, we mention some of the commonly used compounds for oral supplementation in photoprotection and/or skin whitening products with proven efficacy:

- *Polypodium leucotomos* extract (PLE): A widely used extract with antioxidant, immunomodulatory, and photoprotective properties. PLE can significantly reduce erythema, DNA damage, depletion of Langerhans cells, or inflammation induced by photodamage [87, 88]. For this reason, it has been used as an adjunctive treatment for melasma, contributing to improved melasma score indexes or reducing visible light-induced pigmentation [89, 90].

- Pine bark extract, *Pinus pinaster* (PBE): Contains proanthocyanidins, flavonoids, phenolic acids, and other phytoconstituents that scavenge ROS and reduce UV-induced pigmentation. Clinical studies have shown improvements in melasma, general skin tone uniformity, and skin brightness [91, 92].

- Glutathione: As the master endogenous antioxidant molecule in our bodies, glutathione levels are key to keeping excess oxidative stress in check, which can contribute to the appearance of skin dark spots. Clinical studies have shown that oral glutathione might have a benefit in decreasing the melanin index [93, 94]. However, glutathione is poorly absorbed through the oral route, while buccal absorption through sublingual forms is recommended to significantly increase the molecule's systemic bioavailability [95].

- Vitamin C and E: Apart from their proven antioxidant beneficial effects, oral supplementation with these vitamins increases endogenous glutathione levels [96, 97], contributing to the previously mentioned skin brightening effect of glutathione through the systemic route.

- Carotenoids: Members of this family, such as lutein, zeaxanthin, and astaxanthin, have been successfully tested to exhibit a moderate photoprotective effect when combined with topical application [98, 99]

- Tranexamic acid: Despite neither being an antioxidant nor a photoprotector itself, we include tranexamic acid as it is commonly used orally for the control of melasma signs, showing significant efficacy while maintaining a good safety profile [100]. Regarding side effects such as increased blood clots, these appear to be rare, as the dosage used in melasma treatment (around 500 mg/day) is much lower than the required dose to produce hemostasis (2 g). As previously mentioned, its multitarget mechanism of action, from vascular to inflammation regulation, has led to the administration of this ingredient through different routes (oral, topical, mesotherapy) [101]. Interestingly, mesotherapy-applied tranexamic acid has been shown to synergize with vitamin C and glutathione in reducing melasma scores [102].

Noteworthy, the efficacy of some of these compounds is variable depending on the galenic form used for oral supplementation. Some studies have shown that buccal absorption provides higher bioavailability compared to intestinal absorption [95]. Consequently, oral products designed to be absorbed at the buccal level can be a better approach to boost the efficacy of the previously mentioned compounds. In addition, multicomponent formulas, including several of these ingredients, might have synergistic effects on skin photoprotection and whitening effects, which should be considered when choosing the proper product.

Besides the use of oral supplements to reduce systemic oxidative stress and increase photoprotection, dietary patterns must also be taken into consideration. For example, not only can proinflammatory foods trigger a promelanogenic response, but also histamine-rich foods [103, 104]. Histamine links inflammation to pigment production by stimulating melanogenesis through the H2 histamine receptor. Thus, some interventions for skin depigmentation might not work if dietary sources of promelanogenic triggers are not controlled.

7. Multi-step integration and hyperpigmentation management proposal

Because of the observed influences on skin pigmentation, it is clear that hyperpigmentation is a chronic condition, and thus it must be addressed as such. Based on the complex network of pathways, external stimuli, and variables that control skin pigmentation, an effective therapy requires more than isolated interventions. A consistent approach with different steps that cover the key factors in skin melanogenesis and melanin accumulation is essential to obtain visible and successful results. Recent studies based on multi-step protocols, including topical peelings, maintenance depigmenting actives, microneedling and/or laser, and oral antioxidant support, are showing significant positive results in decreasing clinical melasma scores and preventing recurrence [39].

Consequently, we have designed a protocol (see **Figure 1**) that covers a sequentially structured strategy at different time points to target both the causes and consequences of pigment dysregulation, aiming to manage skin hyperpigmentation conditions at its various stages (prevention, correction, treatment). This protocol integrates topical, procedural, and systemic therapies, tailored to the underlying pathophysiological mechanisms and patient-specific factors such as phototype, pigmentation type, and skin sensitivity.

We consider several points to be addressed as part of this approach:

- Synergistic efficacy: Single agents (e.g., TYR inhibitors) often fail due to compensatory melanogenic pathways. Targeting different mechanisms of action from different pathways might exert synergistic effects.

- Reduced resistance: Targeting upstream regulators (e.g., inflammation, ROS) prevents rebound pigmentation.

- UV is the main stimulator of melanogenic pathways, which makes photoprotection a key step in the management of hyperpigmentation conditions.

- Every skin is different: Treatments should be adapted in intensity and duration depending on the skin of the patient, as some skins respond better to treatments while others are more prone to showing adverse reactions to common treatments.

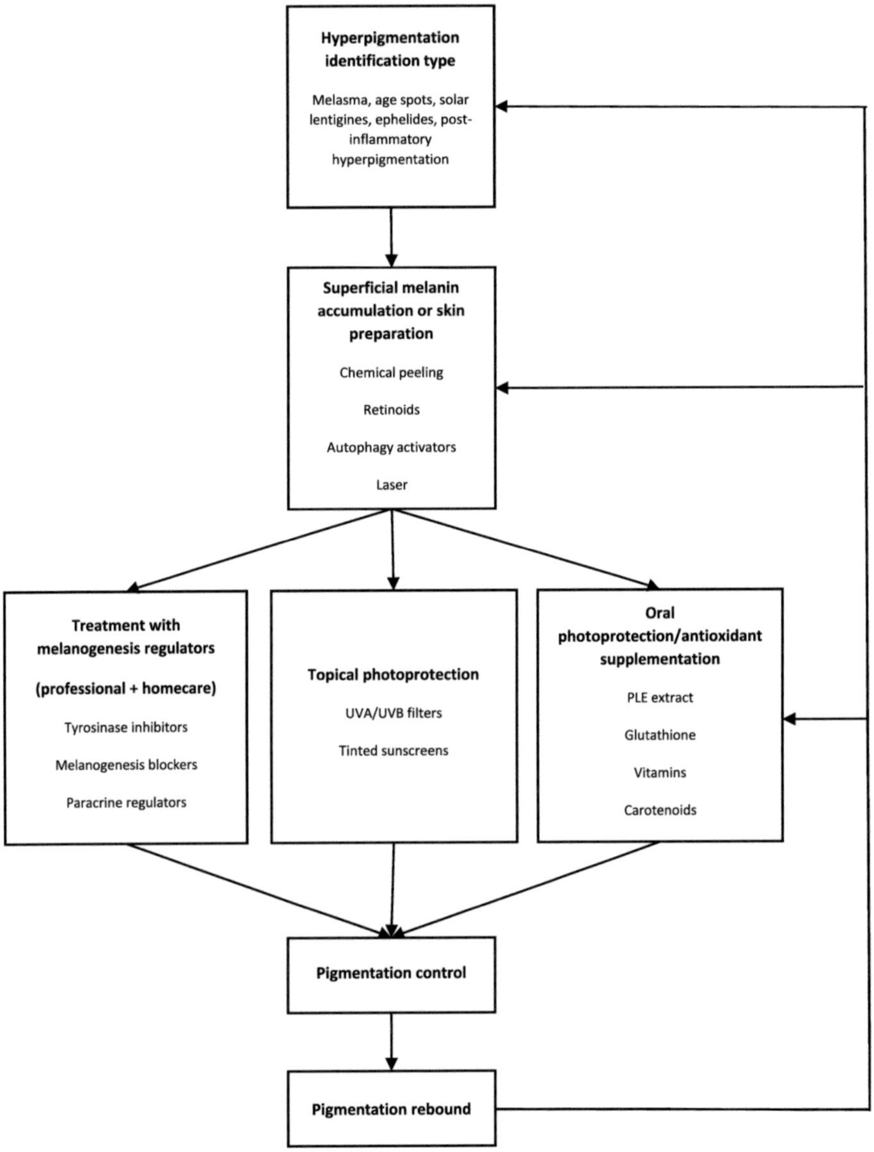

Figure 1.
A scheme describing the multi-step, rationally designed protocol for the successful management of skin hyperpigmentation. Initial steps include the diagnosis of hyperpigmentation conditions to be treated using cosmetic treatments, including those defined in the box. First, accumulated skin in the upper layers of epidermis can be removed using agents that accelerate epidermal turnover and exfoliation. Here, a combination of chemical peelings, retinoids, and autophagy activators offers a good therapeutic solution to effectively remove existing melanin deposits. After this phase, maintenance therapy is based on three main pillars to keep melanocyte activity blocked: (1) the use of melanocyte regulators, including not only inhibitor of melanogenesis activity in the melanocyte but also regulators of proinflammatory paracrine factor release by neighboring cells such as keratinocytes and fibroblasts; (2) topical photoprotection, including both UV and visible light protection, to prevent the triggering of promelanogenic pathways; and (3) oral photoprotection/antioxidant use, which complements topical photoprotection and helps reduce increased systemic oxidative stress levels that typically occur in hyperpigmentation conditions. In the melanocyte-controlling phase, in-cabin whitening treatments performed by clinicians and professional practitioners, combined with homecare products are recommended to maximize the results. When pigmentation rebound occurs due to the chronic characteristic of hyperpigmentation, the treatment approach can be repeated from the previous steps according to the specific needs and features of the pigmentation rebound; diagnosing again the type of hyperpigmentation and either from the melanin removal step or from the maintenance treatment.

- Realistic expectations and patient education: Consistency is key to achieving results, which sometimes might take weeks to months to show a clear improvement. Mild adverse effects, such as irritation or erythema, are expected as treatments are aimed not only at preventing melanin formation but also at removing existing melanin accumulations. Patients should recognize that hyperpigmentation is recurrent, particularly in melasma.

- Systemic health importance: Overall oxidative stress levels in the body can significantly affect skin pigmentation. Also, consider the role of diet, encouraging antioxidant-rich foods, and stress reduction.

Future discoveries regarding the biology of hyperpigmentation and novel therapies will provide additional tools to be integrated into this protocol to further improve melasma control and recurrence. For example, the gut microbiome is widely known to play a key role in many systemic diseases, although its effect on skin hyperpigmentation conditions is almost unknown and is only starting to be characterized [105, 106]. Thus, the influence of microbiome signatures on melasma patients might position the use of probiotics as another complement in multi-step and holistic protocols.

8. Conclusion(s)

Skin hyperpigmentation conditions are a common esthetic issue, and the management of skin hyperpigmentation requires more than a single therapeutic intervention; it demands a comprehensive, multi-step strategy that addresses every stage of pigment formation and persistence. By targeting existing melanin deposits through controlled exfoliation and pigment elimination, inhibiting melanogenesis at its enzymatic and regulatory levels, safeguarding against UV- and visible-light-induced melanocyte stimulation with effective photoprotection, and supporting skin health from within through carefully selected oral supplements, clinicians can achieve more consistent, long-lasting results.

This integrated approach not only enhances treatment efficacy but also reduces the risk of recurrence, a common challenge in pigmentation disorders. Each step of the protocol – whether topical, procedural, nutritional, or preventive – contributes synergistically to the overall outcome. Furthermore, personalizing the regimen based on skin phototype, pigmentation pattern, underlying triggers, and patient lifestyle ensures both safety and adherence.

Ultimately, the success of hyperpigmentation management lies in recognizing it as a chronic, multifactorial condition that requires sustained, coordinated care. By addressing all key mechanisms involved in pigment formation while maintaining ongoing photoprotection and supportive measures, practitioners can offer patients not only visible improvement but also the confidence of long-term pigment control.

Acknowledgments

We would like to thank our colleagues from mesoestetic Pharma Group S.L. and external collaborators who have participated in the product's development, protocol design, and clinical practice for the management of skin hyperpigmentation.

Conflict of Interest

All authors were employed by the company mesoestetic Pharma Group S.L.

Author details

Alfredo Martínez-Gutiérrez*, Neus Calbet-Llopart, Julia Aullo and Mari Carmen González
Mesoestetic Pharma Group S.L., Viladecans, Spain

*Address all correspondence to: amartinez@mesoestetic.com

References

[1] Serre C, Busuttil V, Botto J-M. Intrinsic and extrinsic regulation of human skin melanogenesis and pigmentation. International Journal of Cosmetic Science. 2018;**40**:328–347

[2] Thawabteh AM, Jibreen A, Karaman D, et al. Skin pigmentation types, causes and treatment—a review. Molecules. 2023;**28**. DOI: 10.3390/molecules28124839

[3] Park HY, Kosmadaki M, Yaar M, et al. Cellular mechanisms regulating human melanogenesis. Cellular and Molecular Life Sciences. 2009;**66**:1493–1506

[4] Yuan XH, Jin ZH. Paracrine regulation of melanogenesis. British Journal of Dermatology. 2018;**178**: 632–639

[5] D'Mello S, Finlay G, Baguley B, et al. Signaling pathways in melanogenesis. International Journal of Molecular Sciences 2016;**17**:1144

[6] Lee A-Y. Recent progress in melasma pathogenesis. Pigment Cell & Melanoma Research. 2015;**28**:648–660

[7] Passeron T, Picardo M. Melasma, a photoaging disorder. Pigment Cell & Melanoma Research. 2018;**31**: 461–465

[8] Plensdorf S, Livieratos M, Dada N. Pigmentation disorders: Diagnosis and management. American Family Physician. 2017;**96**:797–804

[9] Shenoy A, Madan R. Post-inflammatory hyperpigmentation: A review of treatment strategies. Journal of Drugs in Dermatology. 2020;**19**: 763–768

[10] Kang HY, Lee JW, Papaccio F, et al. Alterations of the pigmentation system in the aging process. Pigment Cell & Melanoma Research. 2021;**34**:800–813

[11] Espósito ACC, Cassiano DP, da Silva CN, et al. Update on Melasma—Part I: Pathogenesis. Dermatology and Therapy. 2022;**12**:1967–1988

[12] Liu W, Chen Q, Xia Y. New mechanistic insights of Melasma. Clinical, Cosmetic and Investigational Dermatology. 2023;**16**:429–442

[13] Truchuelo M, Cerdá P, Fernández LF. Chemical peeling: A useful tool in the office. Actas Dermo-Sifiliográficas (English Edition). 2017; **108**:315–322

[14] Lee KC, Wambier CG, Soon SL, et al. Basic chemical peeling: Superficial and medium-depth peels. Journal of the American Academy of Dermatology. 2019;**81**:313–324

[15] Sarkar R, Garg V, Bansal S, et al. Comparative evaluation of efficacy and tolerability of glycolic acid, salicylic mandelic acid, and phytic acid combination peels in Melasma. Dermatologic Surgery. 2016;**42**: 384–391

[16] Sahu P, Dayal S, Bhardwaj N. Topical 5% tranexamic acid with 30% glycolic acid peel: An useful combination for accelerating the improvement in melasma. Dermatologic Therapy. 2021;**34**. DOI: 10.1111/dth.15107

[17] Kligman DE, Draelos ZD. Combination superficial peels with salicylic acid and post-peel retinoids.

Journal of Drugs in Dermatology. 2016;**15**:442–50

[18] Joshi SS, Boone SL, Alam M, et al. Effectiveness, safety, and effect on quality of life of topical salicylic acid peels for treatment of postinflammatory hyperpigmentation in dark skin. Dermatologic Surgery. 2009;**35**:638–644

[19] GARG VK, SARKAR R, Agarwal R. Comparative evaluation of beneficiary effects of priming agents (2% hydroquinone and 0.025% retinoic acid) in the treatment of melasma with glycolic acid peels. Dermatologic Surgery. 2008;**34**: 1032–1040

[20] Kalla G, Garg A, Kachhawa D. Chemical peeling--glycolic acid versus trichloroacetic acid in melasma. Indian Journal of Dermatology, Venereology and Leprology. 2001;**67**:82–84

[21] Sharad J. Glycolic acid peel therapy – A current review. Clinical, Cosmetic and Investigational Dermatology. 2013;**6**:281–288

[22] Kucuk OS. Current treatment approaches for Melasma. Bezmialem Science. 2018;**6**:54–62

[23] Cotellessa C, Peris K, Onorati MT, et al. The use of chemical peelings in the treatment of different cutaneous hyperpigmentations. Dermatologic Surgery. 1999;**25**:450–454

[24] Mukherjee S, Date A, Patravale V, et al. Retinoids in the treatment of skin aging: An overview of clinical efficacy and safety. Clinical Interventions in Aging. 2006;**1**:327–348

[25] Riahi RR, Bush AE, Cohen PR. Topical retinoids: Therapeutic mechanisms in the treatment of photodamaged skin. American Journal of Clinical Dermatology. 2016; **17**:265–276

[26] Zasada M, Budzisz E. Retinoids: Active molecules influencing skin structure formation in cosmetic and dermatological treatments. Advances in Dermatology and Allergology. 2019;**36**:392–397

[27] Draelos ZD, Peterson RS. A double-blind, comparative clinical study of newly formulated retinol serums vs tretinoin cream in escalating doses: A method for rapid retinization with minimized irritation. Journal of Drugs in Dermatology. 2020;**19**:625–631

[28] He C, Klionsky DJ. Regulation mechanisms and signaling pathways of autophagy. Annual Review of Genetics. 2009;**43**:67–93

[29] Kim JY, Kim J, Ahn Y, et al. Autophagy induction can regulate skin pigmentation by causing melanosome degradation in keratinocytes and melanocytes. Pigment Cell & Melanoma Research. 2020;**33**:403–415

[30] Chen X, Li M, Li L, et al. Trehalose, sucrose and raffinose are novel activators of autophagy in human keratinocytes through an mTOR-independent pathway. Scientific Reports. 2016;**6**:28423

[31] Jane W, Chen S, Hseu J, et al. The in vitro and in vivo skin-whitening activity of Ectoine through enhanced autophagy in melanocytes and keratinocytes and zebrafish model. BioFactors. 2025;**51**. DOI: 10.1002/biof.70004

[32] Chen S-J, Hseu Y-C, Gowrisankar YV, et al. The anti-melanogenic effects of 3-O-ethyl ascorbic acid via Nrf2-mediated α-MSH

inhibition in UVA-irradiated keratinocytes and autophagy induction in melanocytes. Free Radical Biology and Medicine. 2021;**173**:151–169

[33] Hseu Y-C, Yeh J-T, Vadivalagan C, et al. The in vitro and in vivo depigmentation activity of coenzyme Q0, a major quinone derivative from Antrodia camphorata, through autophagy induction in human melanocytes and keratinocytes. Cell Communication and Signaling. 2024;**22**:151

[34] Hseu Y-C, Vudhya Gowrisankar Y, Wang L-W, et al. The in vitro and in vivo depigmenting activity of pterostilbene through induction of autophagy in melanocytes and inhibition of UVA-irradiated α-MSH in keratinocytes via Nrf2-mediated antioxidant pathways. Redox Biology 2021;**44**:102007

[35] Martínez-Gutiérrez A, Sendros J, Noya T, et al. Apigenin and Phloretin Combination for Skin Aging and Hyperpigmentation Regulation. Cosmetics. 2024;**11**:128

[36] Lee YS, Lee YJ, Lee JM, et al. The low-fluence Q-Switched Nd:YAG laser treatment for Melasma: A systematic review. Medicina (Kaunas, Lithuania). 2022;**58**. DOI: 10.3390/medicina58070936

[37] Tsilika K, Levy JL, Kang HY, et al. A pilot study using reflectance confocal microscopy (RCM) in the assessment of a novel formulation for the treatment of melasma. Journal of Drugs in Dermatology. 2011;**10**:1260–1264

[38] Sarkar R, Kaur C, Bhalla M, et al. The combination of glycolic acid peels with a topical regimen in the treatment of melasma in dark-skinned patients: A comparative study. Dermatologic Surgery. 2002;**28**:828–832

[39] Ravindran J, Suresh A. Effectiveness of a standardised treatment protocol in the management of Melasma: A retrospective analysis. International Journal of Aesthetic Plastic Surgery. 2025;**1**:50–56

[40] Pillaiyar T, Namasivayam V, Manickam M, et al. Inhibitors of melanogenesis: An updated review. Journal of Medicinal Chemistry. 2018;**61**:7395–7418

[41] Zolghadri S, Bahrami A, Hassan Khan MT, et al. A comprehensive review on tyrosinase inhibitors. Journal of Enzyme Inhibition and Medicinal Chemistry. 2019;**34**:279–309

[42] Mann T, Gerwat W, Batzer J, et al. Inhibition of human tyrosinase requires molecular motifs distinctively different from mushroom tyrosinase. Journal of Investigative Dermatology. 2018;**138**:1601–1608

[43] Faloon PW, Bennion M, Weiner WS et al. A Small Molecule Inhibitor of the MITF Molecular Pathway. 2010

[44] Martínez-Gutiérrez A, Bertran A, Noya T, et al. New chalcone-derived molecule for the topical regulation of hyperpigmentation and skin aging. Pharmaceutics. 2024;**16**:1405

[45] Kumari S, Thng S, Verma N, et al. Melanogenesis Inhibitors. Acta Dermato Venereologica. 2018;**98**:924–931

[46] Lee SJ, Son YH, Lee KB, et al. 4-n-butylresorcinol enhances proteolytic degradation of tyrosinase in B16F10 melanoma cells. International Journal of Cosmetic Science. 2017;**39**:248–255

[47] Na J-I, Shin J-W, Choi H-R, et al. Resveratrol as a Multifunctional Topical

Hypopigmenting Agent. International Journal of Molecular Sciences. 2019;**20**. DOI: 10.3390/ijms20040956

[48] Hwang JS, Lee HY, Lim T-Y, et al. Disruption of tyrosinase glycosylation by N-acetylglucosamine and its depigmenting effects in Guinea pig skin and in human skin. Journal of Dermatological Science. 2011;**63**: 199–201

[49] Pan C, Liu X, Zheng Y, et al. The mechanisms of melanogenesis inhibition by glabridin: Molecular docking, PKA/MITF and MAPK/MITF pathways. Food Science and Human Wellness. 2023;**12**:212–222

[50] Lin CB, Babiarz L, Liebel F, et al. Modulation of microphthalmia-associated transcription factor gene expression alters skin pigmentation. Journal of Investigative Dermatology. 2002;**119**:1330–1340

[51] Lee H, Lee W, Chang S, et al. Hesperidin, A popular antioxidant inhibits Melanogenesis via Erk1/2 Mediated MITF degradation. International Journal of Molecular Sciences. 2015;**16**:18384–18395

[52] Noh TK, Chung BY, Kim SY, et al. Novel anti-melanogenesis properties of polydeoxyribonucleotide, a popular wound healing booster. International Journal of Molecular Sciences. 2016;**17**. DOI: 10.3390/ijms17091448

[53] Ito S, Kolbe L, Weets G, et al. Exogenous ochronosis by hydroquinone is not caused by inhibition of homogentisate dioxygenase but potentially by tyrosinase-catalysed metabolism of hydroquinone. British Journal of Dermatology. 2025;**193**: 959–967

[54] Jimbow K, Obata H, Pathak MA, et al. Mechanism of Depigmentation by Hydroquinone. Journal of Investigative Dermatology. 1974;**62**:436–449

[55] Marques C, Hadjab F, Porcello A, et al. Mechanistic Insights into the multiple functions of niacinamide: Therapeutic implications and cosmeceutical applications in functional skincare products. Antioxidants. 2024;**13**:425

[56] Cardinali G, Kovacs D, Picardo M. Mechanisms underlying post-inflammatory hyperpigmentation: Lessons from solar lentigo. Annales de Dermatologie Et de Vénéréologie. 2012;**139**(Suppl 4):S148–152

[57] Imokawa G. Melanocyte activation mechanisms and rational therapeutic treatments of solar lentigos. International Journal of Molecular Sciences. 2019;**20**:3666. DOI: 10.3390/ijms20153666

[58] Alfredo M-G, Maribel P-M, Eloy P-R, et al. Depigmenting topical therapy based on a synergistic combination of compounds targeting the key pathways involved in melasma pathophysiology. Experimental Dermatology. 2023;**32**:611–619

[59] Niwano T, Terazawa S, Nakajima H, et al. Astaxanthin and withaferin A block paracrine cytokine interactions between UVB-exposed human keratinocytes and human melanocytes via the attenuation of endothelin-1 secretion and its downstream intracellular signaling. Cytokine. 2015;**73**:184–197

[60] Nakajima H, Fukazawa K, Wakabayashi Y, et al. Abrogating effect of a xanthophyll carotenoid astaxanthin on the stem cell factor-induced

stimulation of human epidermal pigmentation. Archives of Dermatological Research. 2012;**304**:803–816

[61] Imokawa G, Ishida K. Inhibitors of Intracellular signaling pathways thatlead to stimulated epidermal pigmentation:perspective of anti-pigmenting agents. International Journal of Molecular Sciences. 2014;**15**:8293–8315

[62] Maeda K. Mechanism of action of topical tranexamic acid in the treatment of melasma and sun-induced skin hyperpigmentation. Cosmetics. 2022;**9**:108

[63] Liu L-X, Liao Z-K, Dong B-Q, et al. Tranexamic Acid ameliorates skin hyperpigmentation by downregulating endothelin-1 expression in dermal microvascular endothelial cells. Annals of Dermatology. 2024;**36**:151–162

[64] Kaur S, Kizoulis M, Fantasia J, et al. 4-Hexyl-1,3-phenylenediol, a nuclear factor-κB inhibitor, improves photodamaged skin and clinical signs of ageing in a double-blinded, randomized controlled trial. British Journal of Dermatology. 2015;**173**:218–226

[65] Shariff R, Du Y, Dutta M, et al. Superior even skin tone and anti-ageing benefit of a combination of 4-hexylresorcinol and niacinamide. International Journal of Cosmetic Science. 2022;**44**:103–117

[66] Yokota T, Nishio H, Kubota Y, et al. The inhibitory effect of glabridin from licorice extracts on melanogenesis and inflammation. Pigment Cell Research. 1998;**11**:355–361

[67] Zhang J, Wu X, Zhong B, et al. Review on the diverse biological effects of glabridin. Drug Design, Development and Therapy. 2023;**17**:15–37

[68] Niwano T, Terazawa S, Sato Y, et al. Glucosamine abrogates the stem cell factor + endothelin-1-induced stimulation of melanogenesis via a deficiency in MITF expression due to the proteolytic degradation of CREB in human melanocytes. Archives of Dermatological Research. 2018;**310**:625–637

[69] Zheng H, Pei Q, Yao M. Understanding Melasma: From Pathogenesis to Innovative Treatments. Dermatologic Therapy. 2024;**2024**. DOI: 10.1155/2024/2206130

[70] Ali L, Al Niaimi F. Pathogenesis of Melasma explained. International Journal of Dermatology. 2025;**64**:1201–1212

[71] Flori E, Mastrofrancesco A, Mosca S, et al. Sebocytes contribute to melasma onset. iScience. 2022;**25**:103871

[72] Wu Q, Zheng H, Wu J, et al. The pathogenesis of oxidative stress-induced chloasma and its therapeutic implications. Clinical, Cosmetic and Investigational Dermatology. 2025;**18**:929–947

[73] Geisler AN, Austin E, Nguyen J, et al. Visible light. Part II: Photoprotection against visible and ultraviolet light. Journal of the American Academy of Dermatology. 2021;**84**:1233–1244

[74] Dumbuya H, Grimes P, Lynch S, et al. Impact of iron-oxide containing formulations against visible light-induced skin pigmentation in skin of color individuals. Journal of Drugs in Dermatology. 2020;**19**:712–717

[75] Castanedo-Cazares JP, Hernandez-Blanco D, Carlos-Ortega B, et al.

Near-visible light and UV photoprotection in the treatment of melasma: A double-blind randomized trial. Photodermatology, Photoimmunology & Photomedicine. 2014;**30**:35–42

[76] Sarkar R, Yadav V, Yadav T, et al. Glutathione as a skin-lightening agent and in melasma: A systematic review. International Journal of Dermatology. 2025;**64**:992–1004

[77] Al-Niaimi F, Chiang NYZ. Topical Vitamin C and the Skin: Mechanisms of Action and Clinical Applications. The Journal of Clinical and Aesthetic Dermatology. 2017;**10**:14–17

[78] Kala R, Heiberger N, Mallin H, et al. Reproducible method for assessing the effects of blue light using in vitro human skin tissues. International Journal of Cosmetic Science. 2023;**45**:95–107

[79] Campiche R, Curpen SJ, Lutchmanen-Kolanthan V, et al. Pigmentation effects of blue light irradiation on skin and how to protect against them. International Journal of Cosmetic Science. 2020;**42**:399–406

[80] McDaniel DH, Neudecker BA, DiNardo JC, et al. Clinical efficacy assessment in photodamaged skin of 0.5% and 1.0% idebenone. Journal of Cosmetic Dermatology. 2005;**4**:167–173

[81] Rosic N. Mycosporine-like amino acids: making the foundation for organic personalised sunscreens. Marine Drugs. 2019;**17**:638

[82] Farshi S, Mansouri P. Study of efficacy of microneedling and mesoneedling in the treatment of epidermal melasma: A pilot trial. Journal of Cosmetic Dermatology. 2020;**19**:1093–1098

[83] Rahimi H, Mirnezami M, Yazdabadi A, Hajihashemi A, et al. Evaluation of systemic oxidative stress in patients with melasma. Journal of Cosmetic Dermatology. 2024;**23**: 284–288

[84] Katiyar S, Yadav D, Singh SK. Markers of oxidative stress and tyrosinase activity in Melasma patients: a biochemical investigation. Current Protein & Peptide Science. 2024;**25**: 183–188

[85] Choubey V, Sarkar R, Garg V, et al. Role of oxidative stress in melasma: A prospective study on serum and blood markers of oxidative stress in melasma patients. International Journal of Dermatology. 2017;**56**:939–943

[86] Chen AC, Damian DL, Halliday GM. Oral and systemic photoprotection. Photodermatology, Photoimmunology & Photomedicine. 2014;**30**:102–111

[87] Zattra E, Coleman C, Arad S, et al. Polypodium leucotomos extract decreases UV-Induced Cox-2 expression and inflammation, enhances DNA repair, and decreases mutagenesis in hairless mice. The American Journal of Pathology. 2009;**175**:1952–1961

[88] Villa A, Viera MH, Amini S, et al. Decrease of ultraviolet A light–induced "common deletion" in healthy volunteers after oral Polypodium leucotomos extract supplement in a randomized clinical trial. Journal of the American Academy of Dermatology. 2010;**62**:511–513

[89] Nestor M, Bucay V, Callender V, et al. Polypodium leucotomos as an adjunct treatment of pigmentary disorders. The Journal of Clinical and Aesthetic Dermatology. 2014;**7**:13–17

[90] Mohammad TF, Kohli I, Nicholson CL, et al. Oral polypodium leucotomos extract and its impact on visible light-induced pigmentation in human subjects. Journal of Drugs in Dermatology. 2019;**18**:1198–1203

[91] Grether-Beck S, Marini A, Jaenicke T, et al. French Maritime Pine Bark Extract (Pycnogenol®) effects on human skin: Clinical and molecular evidence. Skin Pharmacology and Physiology. 2016;**29**:13–17

[92] Ni Z, Mu Y, Gulati O. Treatment of melasma with Pycnogenol. Phytotherapy Research. 2002;**16**: 567–571

[93] Arjinpathana N, Asawanonda P. Glutathione as an oral whitening agent: A randomized, double-blind, placebo-controlled study. Journal of Dermatological Treatment. 2012;**23**: 97–102

[94] Weschawalit S, Thongthip S, Phutrakool P, et al. Glutathione and its antiaging and antimelanogenic effects. Clinical, Cosmetic and Investigational Dermatology. 2017;**10**:147–153

[95] Sharma DK, Sharma P. Augmented glutathione absorption from oral mucosa and its effect on skin pigmentation: a clinical review. Clinical, Cosmetic and Investigational Dermatology. 2022;**15**:1853–1862

[96] Costagliola C, Menzione M. Effect of vitamin E on the oxidative state of glutathione in plasma. Clinical Physiology and Biochemistry. 1990;**8**:140–143

[97] Minich DM, Brown BI. A review of dietary (Phyto)nutrients for glutathione support. Nutrients. 2019;**11**:2073. DOI: 10.3390/nu11092073

[98] Palombo P, Fabrizi G, Ruocco V, et al. Beneficial long-term effects of combined oral/topical antioxidant treatment with the carotenoids lutein and zeaxanthin on human skin: A double-blind, placebo-controlled study. Skin Pharmacology and Physiology. 2007;**20**:199–210

[99] Ma Y, Li C, Su W, et al. Carotenoids in skin photoaging: Unveiling protective effects, molecular insights, and safety and bioavailability frontiers. Antioxidants. 2025;**14**:577

[100] Bala HR, Lee S, Wong C, et al. Oral tranexamic acid for the treatment of Melasma: A review. Dermatologic Surgery. 2018;**44**:814–825

[101] Chen Z, Huang L. Different administration routes of tranexamic acid in the treatment of melasma. Chinese Journal of Plastic and Reconstructive Surgery. 2024;**6**:154–158

[102] Iraji F, Nasimi M, Asilian A, et al. Efficacy of mesotherapy with tranexamic acid and ascorbic acid with and without glutathione in treatment of melasma: A split face comparative trial. Journal of Cosmetic Dermatology. 2019;**18**:1416–1421

[103] Zhao Y, Zhang X, Jin H, et al. Histamine Intolerance—A Kind of Pseudoallergic Reaction. Biomolecules. 2022;**12**:454

[104] Yoshida M, Takahashi Y, Inoue S. Histamine induces melanogenesis and morphologic changes by protein kinase a activation via H2 Receptors in human normal melanocytes. Journal of Investigative Dermatology. 2000;**114**:334–342

[105] Liu C, He D, Yu A, et al. Correlation analysis between gut

microbiota characteristics and melasma. Frontiers in Microbiology. 2022;**13**. DOI: 10.3389/fmicb.2022.1051653

[106] Hu Y, Chen Y, Xu J, et al. Dysbiosis of skin microbiome in melasma patients. Pigment Cell & Melanoma Research. 2022;**35**:627–631

Chapter 2

Advances in Melasma Diagnosis and Treatment

Liyuan Zhou, Bingyu Wang, Yiting Zhao, Xidie Yin, Zhi Cao, Shuzhan Shen, Xiuli Wang, Qingyu Zeng and Peiru Wang

Abstract

Melasma is a common acquired hyperpigmentation disorder that primarily affects sun-exposed areas of the face. Recent advances in melasma research have highlighted its complex pathogenesis, involving melanocyte hyperactivity, vascular changes, impaired skin barrier function, and dermal inflammation. Melasma can be accurately diagnosed and classified based on clinical presentation in combination with noninvasive diagnostic tools such as Wood's lamp, dermoscopy, and reflectance confocal microscopy (RCM). Conventional treatments for melasma include systemic and topical medications, chemical peels, phototherapy, and traditional Chinese medicine. In addition, advances in platelet-rich plasma (PRP), microneedling, and nanoparticle-based technology are further enhancing outcomes. Emphasis is also placed on personalized treatment protocols and long-term maintenance strategies to prevent recurrence. This chapter provides a comprehensive overview of current evidence and emerging trends in melasma diagnosis and therapy, serving as a clinical guide for dermatologists and researchers.

Keywords: melasma, hyperpigmentation, pathogenesis, diagnosis, treatment

1. Introduction

Melasma is an acquired pigmentary disorder characterized by irregular brown macules and patches on sun-exposed areas of the face. It results from the excessive deposition of melanin in both the epidermis and dermis. The condition predominantly affects women between 30 and 40 years of age, particularly those with Fitzpatrick skin types III and IV. Approximately 48% of patients have a family history of melasma, with 97% of these involving first-degree relatives [1]. Various factors may contribute to the onset of melasma, such as ultraviolet radiation, genetic predisposition, and hormonal influences. The pathophysiology of melasma is complex. Although it was initially thought to involve only melanocytes, recent studies suggest that its development is associated with interactions among keratinocytes, fibroblasts, mast cells, abnormal gene regulation, increased angiogenesis, and disruption of the basement membrane [2, 3].

1.1 Clinical subtypes

Clinically, melasma can be classified according to vascular involvement, pigment depth, and anatomical distribution. Based on vascular involvement, it is categorized as either the melanotic type or the vascularized-melanotic type. According to pigment location, it is classified into the epidermal type, characterized by epidermal hyperpigmentation, and the mixed type, which involves a combination of epidermal pigmentation and superficial dermal melanocyte deposition. Notably, these classifications provide important guidance for predicting treatment responses. Based on the anatomical distribution of skin lesions, melasma is further subdivided into three distribution patterns: centrofacial, malar, and mandibular types [4].

1.2 Impact on quality of life

Melasma is a chronic skin disorder requiring long-term management, which adds to the cumulative burden on patients' quality of life. According to the SKINDEX-16 and MELASQOL instruments, the aspects of life most affected by melasma include social interaction, leisure activities, and emotional well-being. Other domains, such as sexual relationships, occupational functioning, and family dynamics, are also impacted to varying degrees. Notably, the severity of melasma—as assessed by the Melasma Area and Severity Index (MASI)—is only moderately correlated with patients' self-reported quality of life ($r = 0.30$), indicating a potential disconnect between clinical severity and psychological burden. Patients with underlying psychological or emotional disturbances and those using skin-bleaching creams report significantly higher MELASQOL scores, suggesting that psychosocial factors play a substantial role in quality of life [5].

The translation and validation of the MELASQOL scale among Latin American populations in Southern Brazil have demonstrated its broad applicability and potential for widespread clinical use. Additionally, patients with lower educational attainment (≤6th grade) exhibited higher MELASQOL scores compared to those with higher education levels (≥7th grade) (49.4 vs. 39.3, $P < 0.05$), and those with longer disease duration reported significantly worse scores (47.7 vs. 35.5, $P < 0.05$) [6–8].

These findings support the inclusion of validated quality-of-life instruments such as MELASQOL in clinical guidelines to inform treatment decisions and assess prognosis. Approximately one-third of patients reported changes in their sun protection habits following diagnosis, reflecting the disease's persistent influence on daily behavior [1]. Significant improvements in quality-of-life scores have been observed in patients treated with oral tranexamic acid (TXA) combined with hydroquinone (HQ), and similar benefits have been reported in those receiving polysaccharide peptide therapy, indicating that effective pigmentation reduction is associated with improved quality of life.

2. Risk factors and pathogenesis of melasma

2.1 Risk factors

The risk factors of melasma include positive family history, sun exposure and hormonal fluctuations. Ultraviolet (UV) radiation contributes to the initiation and progression of melasma through multiple pathways. Hormonal influences, including those arising from pregnancy, oral contraceptive use, prostate cancer treatment, and hormone replacement therapy, have been associated with the onset or aggravation of melasma, suggesting that estrogen and progesterone play significant roles in its pathogenesis [9, 10]. Lesional areas in melasma exhibit features consistent with chronic photodamage. UV-induced damage is believed to contribute to a pathological cycle of photoaging, disruption of the dermal microenvironment, and persistent pigmentation, thereby accelerating disease progression [11].

2.1.1 Positive family history

Between 41 and 61% of melasma patients have a family history of the condition among first-degree relatives—significantly higher than the general population's incidence of 16 to 28%. Emerging evidence suggests that melasma may follow an autosomal dominant inheritance pattern. In genetically predisposed individuals, the expression of genes involved in melanin synthesis, hormone receptor regulation, and oxidative stress responses is often upregulated, whereas the expression of related DNA repair genes appears downregulated [11].

2.1.2 Solar radiation

UV radiation induces melasma *via* two primary mechanisms: direct damage to the basement membrane and increased melanin synthesis through various signaling pathways. Chronic exposure to UVA and high-energy visible light (HEVL) leads to structural alterations in the basement membrane, characterized by thinning, discontinuities, loss of anchoring fibrils, and the presence of pendulous melanocytes [12].

UV radiation promotes tyrosinase expression by upregulating microphthalmia-associated transcription factor (MITF), which binds to the TYR gene promoter and regulates the expression of other melanogenic enzymes, such as tyrosinase-related protein-1 (TRP-1) and TRP-2. Additionally, UV activates melanocortin-1 receptor (MC1R), enhancing MITF activity through the cAMP–PKA signaling pathway, ultimately increasing melanin synthesis. The Val92Met polymorphism of MC1R has been significantly associated with an increased risk of melasma in South Asian populations [9].

Unlike UV radiation, blue-violet light (415–465 nm) stimulates melanocytes by activating calcium-dependent signaling *via* the photoreceptor opsin 3 (OPN3). This triggers a signaling cascade involving intracellular calcium influx, CAMKII activation, and phosphorylation of CREB, ERK, and p38, ultimately leading to enhanced MITF activity and upregulation of TYR and dopachrome tautomerase (DCT) expression [13].

2.1.3 Hormone fluctuations

Estrogen significantly increases PDZK1 expression, contributing to melanin synthesis. In both monoculture and co-culture systems of melanocytes and keratinocytes, estrogen treatment at concentrations of 10–100 nM has been shown to elevate PDZK1 protein levels in a dose-dependent manner. This regulatory pattern aligns with that observed in other estrogen receptor-positive cells (e.g., breast cancer cells), where the NHERF protein family is also modulated. The estrogen–PDZK1 pathway stimulates melanogenesis by enhancing tyrosinase activity and modulating ion transporters involved in melanin regulation [14].

2.2 Pathogenesis

2.2.1 Increased melanin synthesis

Melanocytes express Wnt inhibitory factor-1 (WIF-1) under both *in vivo* and *in vitro* conditions. WIF-1 modulates melanocyte activity through three major pathways: (1) a β-catenin-dependent pathway, in which inhibition of GSK3β stabilizes β-catenin, leading to its nuclear translocation and subsequent activation of MITF transcription; (2) direct regulation *via* increased gene expression and paracrine stimulation of MITF and tyrosinase; and (3) stromal cell-derived WIF-1 that activates melanocytes remotely. Nuclear localization of β-catenin in certain melanocytes further suggests that the WIF-1/β-catenin/MITF axis plays a critical role in pathological pigmentation [15].

In melasma, WIF-1 expression is reduced, whereas Wnt-1 and Wnt-5a levels are elevated, indicating that hyperactivation of the Wnt signaling pathway is a hallmark of the disease. Both canonical and non-canonical Wnt pathways are variably upregulated in patients, and Wnt signaling indirectly promotes pigmentation *via* paracrine interactions between keratinocytes, fibroblasts, and melanocytes. Regulatory molecules such as sFRP2 and Wnt5a synergistically amplify this signaling. Notably, UV radiation does not alter WIF-1 levels, suggesting that Wnt pathway dysregulation is not solely attributable to photodamage [15, 16].

2.2.2 Vascularity influence melanogenesis

Melasma lesions are characterized by elevated epidermal vascular endothelial growth factor (VEGF) expression, increased dermal vascularity, and visible capillary dilation with erythema. VEGF is implicated in both melanogenesis and vascular proliferation. Functional VEGF receptors (VEGFRs) are expressed on melanocytes, and stimulation by VEGF165 activates these receptors, upregulating melanin-related proteins such as MITF, tyrosinase, TRP-1, and TRP-2 [17].

Endothelin-1 (EDN1), secreted by microvascular endothelial cells, binds to its receptor EDNRB and activates the MAPK/ERK/p38 signaling cascade, thereby stimulating melanin synthesis. EDN1 also synergizes with the MITF pathway to enhance tyrosinase expression. Additionally, inducible nitric oxide synthase (iNOS) is upregulated in melasma lesions, and nitric oxide (NO) produced by vascular endothelium further promotes MITF expression and melanogenesis [18].

2.2.3 Inflammation enhance melanosome transportaion

Transcriptomic studies have demonstrated significant upregulation of interleukin-6 receptor (IL-6R) and endothelin-1 receptor (ET-1R) expression in the basal layer of melasma lesions compared to adjacent normal skin. ET-1R expression is predominantly localized to the basal layer, while IL-6R is upregulated throughout the entire epidermis. IL-6 promotes dendritic cell differentiation, and ET-1 activates melanocytes *via* EDNRB, resulting in more elaborate and branched dendritic processes. These morphological changes imply enhanced melanosome transport to adjacent keratinocytes, contributing to increased pigmentation. This inflammation upregulation is also observed in other pigmentary disorders, such as solar lentigines and acne, suggesting a shared pathophysiological mechanism in facial hyperpigmentation [19, 20].

2.2.4 Impaired skin barrier function

The stratum corneum in melasma-affected skin is notably thinner, with impaired barrier function reflected by increased transepidermal water loss and delayed barrier recovery. Concurrently, matrix metalloproteinase (MMP-2 and MMP-9) activity is elevated, contributing to the degradation of type IV and type VII collagen. These changes reduce the skin's resilience to environmental stimuli and compromise its protective functions [10, 11].

2.2.5 Other contributing factors

Chronic diseases, medication use, cosmetic products, thyroid dysfunction, and vitamin D deficiency have all been identified as contributing factors in melasma pathogenesis [21, 22].

In summary, the pathogenesis of melasma is multifactorial and involves interconnected biological pathways. These include pigmentation, vascular changes, inflammation, barrier dysfunction, and external or systemic factors. Ongoing research continues to elucidate new molecular targets and deepen understanding of this complex condition.

3. Diagnosis and differential diagnosis

Melasma can be comprehensively diagnosed based on the patient's medical history and characteristic clinical manifestations. In combination with noninvasive diagnostic tools such as Wood's lamp, VISIA digital facial imaging system, dermoscopy, reflectance confocal microscopy (RCM), Chromameter, and Mexameter, melasma can be diagnosis and classified precisely.

3.1 Advances in the application of noninvasive skin imaging techniques in the diagnosis of melasma

3.1.1 Wood's lamp

Wood's lamp is the most commonly used auxiliary tool in the diagnosis of melasma, primarily employed to assess the depth of pigment deposition [23]. When the pigmentation is located in the epidermis, the lesions typically appear as brown patches under clinical observation, and show accentuated pigmentation with well-defined borders under Wood's lamp examination. In contrast, when the pigmentation is situated in the dermis, the lesions clinically appear bluish-gray or blue, and exhibit little to no enhancement in color with poorly defined margins under Wood's lamp illumination [24].

Wood's lamp is inexpensive and easy to use; however, it has limited diagnostic accuracy. It provides only subjective and rough assessments, lacks objective quantifiable data, and is unable to visualize vascular features or support longitudinal monitoring.

3.1.2 VISIA digital skin imaging analysis system

The VISIA imaging system captures highly standardized photographs, facilitating consistent monitoring of disease progression. Utilizing RBX technology, it provides a comprehensive assessment of skin pigmentation, including melanin deposition and vascular dilation. Compared to Wood's lamp, VISIA demonstrates higher concordance with dermoscopic and histopathological findings. Furthermore, it generates objective quantitative data that reflect the degree of pigmentation and vascular changes. These output values show strong correlation with the Melasma Area and Severity Index (MASI), making VISIA a valuable tool for the auxiliary diagnosis, classification, treatment planning, and follow-up of melasma [18].

3.1.3 Dermoscopy

Dermoscopy is a commonly used noninvasive diagnostic tool for pigmented skin disorders. In melasma, typical dermoscopic features include light to dark brown pigmentation, with pseudo-network, annular, and arcuate structures observed under magnification [25]. A characteristic dermoscopic finding in melasma is a pseudo-network of pigmentation, with relative sparing of perifollicular and adnexal areas. This feature aids in differentiating melasma from other disorders such as lichen planus pigmentosus, pigmented contact dermatitis, and exogenous ochronosis [26]. In terms of classification, epidermal melasma is suggested by light brown patches with well-defined borders and network or globular patterns, whereas dermal melasma is characterized by poorly defined gray or bluish patches with dot-like, annular, or crescent-shaped structures—features typically associated with more treatment-resistant cases. Compared to Wood's lamp, dermoscopy provides superior visualization of both pigmentation depth and dermal vasculature, contributing to more accurate classification, therapeutic decision-making, and prognostic evaluation [27].

In addition, dermoscopy allows clear visualization of capillary dilation (**Figure 1**). This facilitates not only the classification and monitoring of treatment response, but also serves as a baseline evaluation before initiating topical corticosteroid therapy. It may help in detecting adverse effects such as telangiectasia induced by long-term corticosteroid use, and in identifying patients most likely to respond to vascular-targeting agents such as tranexamic acid [28].

3.1.4 Reflectance confocal microscopy (RCM)

RCM utilizes an 830 nm laser beam to perform optical sectioning and imaging of cells and tissues, enabling high-resolution, *in vivo* visualization of skin morphology

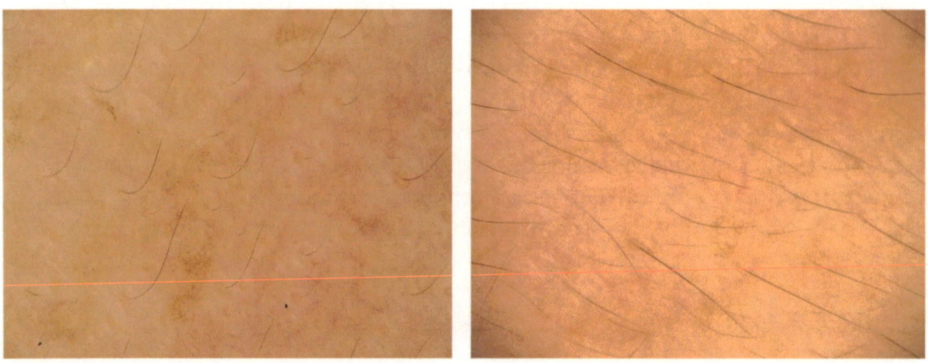

Figure 1.
Dermoscopic examination revealed brown pigmentation and capillary dilation.

at the cellular level, particularly in the epidermis and superficial dermis. In melasma lesions, RCM reveals a highly refractile cobblestone pattern in the basal layer of the epidermis, corresponding to pigment-laden basal keratinocytes observed in histopathological sections [29]. In addition, highly refractile dendritic melanocytes can be observed in the basal layer and at the dermoepidermal junction (**Figure 2**). In progressive stages of the disease, active melanocytes with dendritic and starburst-like morphology are frequently detected, and melanin granules may also be present in the superficial dermis [30]. Moreover, the presence of moderately refractile mononuclear cell infiltration in the dermis can be used to assess inflammatory activity. RCM also allows for semiquantitative evaluation of both pigmentation and inflammatory infiltrates, making it a useful tool for objective efficacy assessment. Therefore, RCM holds great potential for the diagnosis, classification, staging, treatment guidance, and therapeutic monitoring of melasma [29].

3.1.5 Spectrophotometric devices: Chromameter and mexameter

The Chromameter (CR200 and CR400) and Mexameter (MX16 and MX18) are two commonly used noninvasive instruments for assessing skin pigmentation. Compared with the MASI, which is relatively subjective and involves complex calculations, these devices enable quantitative evaluation of color changes in lesions before and after treatment, and are frequently used to assess the severity and therapeutic efficacy of melasma [31]. The Chromameter uses the CIE Lab* color space to analyze light reflected from the skin surface at wavelengths of 450 nm (blue), 560 nm (green), and 600 nm (red). In this system, L* represents lightness (ranging from 0 for black to 100 for white), primarily reflecting melanin levels; a* represents the red-green axis (ranging from −60 to +60), mainly indicating hemoglobin content.

The Mexameter emits light at specific wavelengths—568 nm (green), 660 nm (red), and 880 nm (infrared)—and calculates the intensity of light absorption and reflection to derive the melanin index (M) and erythema index (E). The M value is calculated based on red and infrared absorption, while the E value is derived from green and red light absorption. Both instruments show good correlation when

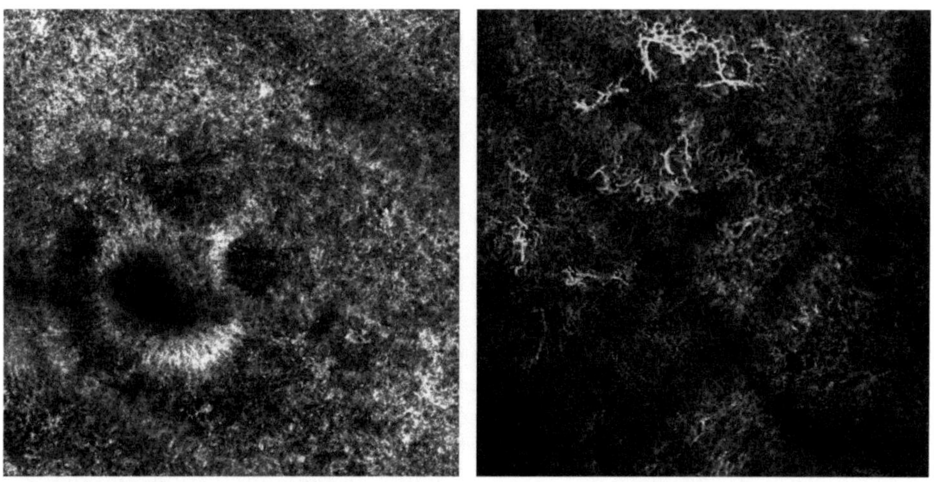

Figure 2.
Highly refractile dendritic melanocytes were observed in the basal layer and superficial dermis.

measuring normal skin color. However, compared with the Mexameter's E value, the Chromameter's a* value is more sensitive to changes in erythema. Conversely, the L* value from the Chromameter, which reflects skin brightness, may be influenced by erythema and is thus less specific than the M value in reflecting melanin content. This is particularly relevant in erythematous skin, where the M value provides a more specific assessment of melanin [32].

3.2 Differential diagnosis

Melasma should be differentiated from other pigmented skin conditions such as freckles, nevus of Ota, Hori's Nevus, pigmented contact dermatitis, and post-inflammatory hyperpigmentation.

3.2.1 Nevus of Ota

Nevus of Ota typically presents at birth or shortly thereafter and is clinically characterized by unilateral, confluent bluish patches located on the zygomatic and temporal regions, as well as the conjunctiva. Under RCM, melanin content in the basal layer of the epidermis is generally normal, while the mid-dermis shows a moderate number of highly refractile dendritic melanocytes or irregular clusters of hyper-refractive melanocytes [33].

3.2.2 Hori's nevus

This condition commonly affects young women in their 20s to 30s and is characterized clinically by symmetrically distributed, round, scattered, non-confluent bluish-gray macules on the bilateral zygomatic and temporal regions. RCM findings reveal normal melanin levels in the basal epidermis, with scattered, slender, hyper-refractive dendritic melanocytes observed between collagen fiber bundles in the superficial to mid-dermis [33].

3.2.3 Post-inflammatory hyperpigmentation (PIH)

PIH refers to light brown, violaceous-brown, or dark brown patches that develop secondary to acute or chronic inflammatory dermatoses, confined to areas of previous inflammation. These lesions have well-defined borders. Diagnosis is primarily based on a history of prior inflammatory skin disease followed by the onset of pigmentation.

4. Advances in treatment

The treatment of melasma is guided by several core principles, including the inhibition of melanogenesis, anti-inflammatory effects, suppression of angiogenesis, restoration of the skin barrier, and prevention of photoaging. The therapeutic goals are to lighten or eliminate hyperpigmented lesions, reduce their size or achieve complete resolution, and minimize recurrence. Specific treatment approaches include the avoidance of triggering factors, implementation of photoprotection, and the use of functional skincare products aimed at restoring the skin barrier and promoting depigmentation. Based on clinical staging and classification, a comprehensive treatment strategy often involves a combination of systemic and topical medications, phototherapy, traditional Chinese medicine (TCM), and other integrative therapies.

4.1 Systemic therapy

4.1.1 Tranexamic acid

Tranexamic acid (TXA) is a synthetic lysine analog with antifibrinolytic properties. It inhibits melanogenesis primarily by modulating the plasminogen–plasmin pathway, thereby disrupting the interaction between keratinocytes and melanocytes [34]. In addition to its effects on pigment regulation, TXA also exhibits anti-angiogenic activity and suppresses mast cell activation. These properties make it particularly advantageous for treating vascular-type melasma characterized by capillary dilation as observed *via* RCM or dermoscopy, as well as melasma with inflammatory cell infiltration [35, 36]. TXA can be administered through various routes, including topical application, microneedling-assisted delivery, mesotherapy, and systemic administration. Among these, topical application is the most commonly used due to its favorable tolerability and demonstrated efficacy in vascular-type melasma [37]. Novel topical formulations such as TXA liposomes and TXA patch preparations have been developed to enhance transdermal absorption, improve skin hydration, and reduce irritation [38]. Microneedling or intradermal injection of TXA allows for higher drug concentration in the dermis, making it particularly suitable for dermal or mixed-type melasma [39, 40]. Oral TXA, typically administered at a daily dose of 500–1000 mg, has been shown to improve melasma severity and modulate systemic inflammation. It is considered a safe and effective option for refractory melasma, although potential side effects include gastrointestinal discomfort and menstrual irregularities [28, 41]. Despite the availability of multiple administration routes and promising results, recurrence remains a major therapeutic challenge. Therefore, more effective and sustainable treatment strategies are needed to alleviate the impact of melasma on patients' quality of life and psychosocial well-being [34].

4.1.2 Vitamin C

Vitamin C plays a beneficial role in the treatment of melasma through its antioxidant properties and its ability to inhibit tyrosinase activity. It directly reduces melanin synthesis by suppressing tyrosinase activity, and indirectly protects the skin by neutralizing free radicals generated by UV radiation and environmental pollutants, thereby preventing oxidative stress, minimizing free radical–induced skin damage, and ultimately decreasing melanin production [42, 43]. In addition, vitamin C can be used in combination with other agents such as tranexamic acid and glutathione to enhance its therapeutic efficacy against melasma.

4.1.3 Vitamin E

Vitamin E is a fat-soluble vitamin with multiple biological functions, including antioxidant activity, inhibition of tyrosinase activity, suppression of melanin transfer, and anti-inflammatory effects. It interferes with lipid peroxidation of the melanocyte membrane and increases intracellular glutathione levels, thereby helping to protect skin cells from free radical–induced damage and reducing pigmentation caused by oxidative stress [44, 45]. Additionally, vitamin E decreases the production of inflammatory mediators, contributing to the alleviation of inflammation-related symptoms in melasma [45]. It is commonly used in combination with other therapeutic agents or antioxidants, such as vitamin C, to enhance treatment efficacy [44].

4.1.4 Other antioxidants

Other antioxidants include glycyrrhizic acid and glutathione. Glycyrrhizic acid exerts anti-inflammatory effects by inhibiting mast cell degranulation and reducing the production of inflammatory mediators such as leukotrienes. Glutathione, on the other hand, inhibits melanogenesis by binding the thiol group of its molecule to copper ions at the active site of tyrosinase, thereby suppressing its enzymatic activity. It can be administered orally or intravenously, and is often used in combination with vitamin C to enhance its depigmenting effect [46].

4.2 Topical agents

4.2.1 Hydroquinone and its combination formulations

Hydroquinone (HQ) and its combination formulations remain the first-line topical therapy for melasma [47]. The primary mechanism of HQ involves the competitive inhibition of tyrosinase activity and the promotion of melanosome degradation. The triple combination (TC) therapy—comprising hydroquinone, a corticosteroid, and a retinoid—has been shown to enhance efficacy while reducing cutaneous irritation [48]. Additionally, the use of platelet-rich plasma (PRP) in combination with 4% hydroquinone has demonstrated significant improvement in both the area and severity of melasma, as measured by the MASI [49]. These combination formulations have consistently exhibited favorable efficacy and safety profiles in clinical treatment. During hydroquinone therapy, regular dermoscopic monitoring is recommended to detect adverse reactions early. The appearance of homogeneous brown patches without a pseudo-reticular pigment network under dermoscopy may indicate exogenous ochronosis, in which case hydroquinone should be promptly discontinued.

4.2.2 Arbutin

Arbutin is a naturally derived compound extracted from plants, primarily composed of α-arbutin and β-arbutin. It functions as a tyrosinase inhibitor, thereby reducing melanin production. In addition to its depigmenting effect, arbutin also exhibits anti-inflammatory, antimicrobial, and moisturizing properties. These characteristics contribute to alleviating skin inflammation, preventing post-inflammatory hyperpigmentation, and promoting skin repair and regeneration [50]. Studies have shown that topical formulations containing 5% α-arbutin and 2% kojic acid demonstrate comparable efficacy to triple combination cream (TCC) in the treatment of melasma [51].

4.2.3 Asiaticoside

Asiaticoside is a triterpenoid compound extracted from *Centella asiatica*. Similar to arbutin, it exhibits multiple biological activities, including tyrosinase inhibition, anti-inflammatory and antioxidant effects, as well as the promotion of skin repair.

4.2.4 Retinoids

Topical retinoids, typically in the form of 0.05 to 0.1% creams or gels, are commonly applied once nightly for a treatment duration of approximately 6 months. Adverse effects may include skin dryness, erythema, pruritus, and a burning sensation. Retinoids are primarily indicated for epidermal-type melasma.

4.2.5 Azelaic acid

Azelaic acid is usually administered as a 15 to 20% cream applied twice daily for about 6 months. Adverse reactions occur in 1–5% of patients and may include itching, burning, stinging, and numbness; less than 1% of patients may experience erythema, dryness, scaling, or even contact dermatitis. It is mainly suitable for treating epidermal-type melasma.

4.3 Chemical peels

Chemical peeling is considered a second-line treatment for moderate-to-severe melasma, primarily targeting the epidermal component of the condition. Commonly used peeling agents include glycolic acid, salicylic acid, and trichloroacetic acid [52]. For patients with epidermal-type melasma—characterized by epidermal pigmentation as indicated by dermoscopy or RCM—chemical peels can be applied during the stable phase, in conjunction with basic therapy and topical and/or oral medications. This approach accelerates epidermal turnover and promotes the elimination of melanin-laden keratinocytes and melanin deposits [53, 54]. Additionally, chemical peeling disrupts intercellular junctions between keratinocytes, enhancing the permeability of the skin and facilitating the penetration of topical agents. Therefore, when combined with topical medications, chemical peels may enhance overall treatment efficacy [55].

4.4 Phototherapy and laser-based treatments

Phototherapy is considered a third-line treatment for refractory melasma, particularly in patients who show poor response to topical agents or chemical peels. It should only be administered during the stable phase of the disease. RCM can be employed to confirm disease stability by identifying specific features, such as a reduction in dendritic and starburst-like melanocytes in the basal epidermal layer and a decreased presence of mononuclear inflammatory cells in the superficial dermis. The selection of appropriate phototherapeutic devices and parameters should be guided by the specific pathophysiological features observed through imaging techniques. For example, if RCM or dermoscopy reveals dilated dermal blood vessels, or if vascular imaging with VISIA indicates prominent telangiectasia, intense pulsed light (IPL) and pulsed dye laser (PDL) may be considered as suitable options. Furthermore, if RCM detects a large number of polygonal or poorly defined round hyper-refractive structures (melanin-laden macrophages) between dermal collagen bundles, or dermoscopy suggests dermal-type melasma, phototherapy may be effective in targeting the persistent dermal pigmentation.

4.4.1 Red and yellow light

Red and yellow light therapy has emerged as a noninvasive adjunctive modality in the management of melasma. Red light (wavelengths around 630–660 nm) penetrates into the dermis and exerts anti-inflammatory and collagen-stimulating effects, which may help improve skin texture and reduce post-inflammatory hyperpigmentation. Yellow light (wavelengths around 570–590 nm) is primarily absorbed by superficial skin layers and blood vessels, promoting lymphatic drainage, reducing erythema, and modulating melanogenesis through anti-inflammatory and vascular-targeted mechanisms [56].

4.4.2 IPL and PDL

IPL and PDL have demonstrated significant therapeutic effects on dermal vasculature. Studies have shown that, following treatment, the expression of vascular endothelial growth factor (VEGF) in lesional skin is markedly reduced, accompanied by a decrease in the number of blood vessels [57, 58]. The advantage of IPL lies in its broad wavelength spectrum (400–1200 nm), which allows for variable penetration depths and enables absorption by multiple chromophores in the skin, including melanin, hemoglobin, and water. This enables IPL to target both epidermal and dermal melanin, as well as dermal vasculature, while simultaneously stimulating collagen production and promoting dermal remodeling. Therefore, IPL is considered a favorable treatment option for melasma associated with vascular dilation and for treatment-resistant mixed-type melasma. PDL primarily targets dermal blood vessels and is suitable for vascular-type melasma. When combined with low-fluence Q-switched Nd: YAG laser, PDL has been shown to significantly reduce MASI scores and improve dermal vascular dilation in affected patients [59].

4.4.3 Low-fluence Q-switched Nd: YAG laser

The Q-switched laser delivers pulses in the nanosecond range, significantly shorter than the thermal relaxation time of melanosomes. This allows for selective photothermolysis of melanosomes with minimal collateral damage to surrounding tissues, making it widely used in the treatment of hyperpigmentary disorders [60]. The large-spot, low-fluence (1.6–3.8 J/cm^2, spot size 6–7 mm) Q-switched Nd: YAG 1064 nm laser specifically targets melanosomes while minimizing injury to melanocytes and keratinocytes. This subcellular-level mechanism of action makes it a commonly used modality for melasma treatment. It is typically administered once every 4 weeks, with a standard course comprising approximately 10 sessions, and is generally well tolerated by patients [60, 61]. Studies have shown that after treatment with the Q-switched Nd: YAG 1064 nm laser, melanocytes in the lesional area exhibit reduced cell volume and shortened or absent dendritic processes. However, adverse effects such as punctate hypopigmentation may occur. To minimize these risks, pre-treatment imaging with a Wood's lamp or VISIA UV photography is recommended to enable early detection of pigmentary changes [62].

4.4.4 Picosecond laser

Compared to Q-switched lasers, picosecond lasers have a shorter pulse duration, resulting in significantly reduced thermal effects and enhanced mechanical effects. This allows for the use of lower energy levels to instantaneously disrupt melanin particles without damaging surrounding cells, thereby facilitating more precise subcellular-level treatment. Picosecond lasers are characterized by rapid efficacy and minimal side effects in the treatment of melasma. A comparative study between

755 nm picosecond laser and 1064 nm Nd: YAG laser demonstrated that patients showed marked improvement after a single picosecond laser session, with significantly better outcomes observed after four treatments in the picosecond laser group [63]. Additionally, picosecond lasers can induce laser-induced optical breakdown (LIOB), which improves the dermal-epidermal junction (DEJ) and promotes regeneration of the dermal extracellular matrix (ECM). This process transiently opens epidermal channels, enhancing the immediate absorption of topically applied agents, such as tranexamic acid and other whitening compounds, thereby achieving synergistic effects [64].

4.4.5 Fractional laser

Fractional laser technology divides a large laser spot into numerous smaller microspots, ensuring that only a fraction of the skin is treated during each session. This preserves a substantial amount of intact skin, thereby accelerating post-treatment healing, reducing inflammatory responses, and minimizing the risks of scarring and post-inflammatory hyperpigmentation. Fractional lasers are classified into ablative and non-ablative types based on whether the epidermis is disrupted. Non-ablative fractional lasers effectively stimulate regeneration of the epidermis, dermal-epidermal junction (DEJ), and dermis without compromising epidermal integrity, resulting in minimal trauma and making them suitable for melasma treatment [65]. Compared with intense pulsed light (IPL) and Q-switched lasers, fractional lasers offer sustained skin rejuvenation effects lasting 3–6 months. Additionally, the microchannels created by fractional lasers serve as efficient drug delivery pathways, a technique known as laser-assisted drug delivery (LADD) [66]. Studies have demonstrated that immediate topical application of tranexamic acid solution (4 mg/ml) following low-fluence CO_2 fractional laser treatment enhances tranexamic acid absorption, leading to a significant reduction in modified Melasma Area and Severity Index (mMASI) scores. The therapeutic efficacy is comparable to microneedling injections, with patients experiencing no significant discomfort or post-inflammatory hyperpigmentation [67].

4.5 Emerging therapies

4.5.1 Platelet-rich plasma (PRP)

Platelet-rich plasma (PRP), a commonly utilized treatment in various dermatologic conditions, has emerged as a viable option for addressing melasma in recent years [68]. Its effectiveness in melasma treatment lies in its ability to inhibit melanin synthesis through delayed extracellular signal-regulated kinase activation [69]. Studies have shown that treatment with platelet-rich plasma (PRP) significantly reduces the area and severity of melasma, as indicated by decreased modified Melasma Area and Severity Index (mMASI) scores [70].

4.5.2 Microneedle injection

Microneedle injection enhances transdermal drug delivery by creating microchannels in the skin, thereby improving therapeutic efficacy. Studies have shown that microneedles significantly increase drug permeability, particularly in pigmented areas at the epidermal–dermal junction [71]. This technique not only elevates local drug concentration but also reduces systemic side effects [72]. Evidence indicates that combining microneedle injection with pharmacological agents—such as tranexamic acid, kojic acid, and retinol—yields superior outcomes compared to monotherapy or laser treatment alone [73]. Moreover, microneedle injection can be effectively combined with other therapeutic modalities, such as chemical peels and laser therapies, to further enhance clinical efficacy [71].

4.5.3 Nanoparticle-based technologies

In recent years, nanoparticle-based technologies have garnered increasing attention in the treatment of melasma. By enhancing transdermal drug delivery and improving targeting capabilities, these technologies offer novel strategies for melasma management. Recent studies have introduced a nanotechnology-based tranexamic acid microemulsion that demonstrates therapeutic efficacy comparable to that of laser or microneedle-assisted therapies, with a superior safety profile. Moreover, as a noninvasive approach, nanoemulsions eliminate the need for invasive procedures such as laser or microneedling, while simultaneously enhancing drug penetration efficiency [74].

4.6 Traditional Chinese medicine treatment

In traditional Chinese medicine (TCM), melasma is categorized based on its pathogenesis into patterns such as liver qi stagnation, qi stagnation with blood stasis, spleen and stomach deficiency, and liver-kidney deficiency. Treatment strategies typically involve soothing the liver, strengthening the spleen, tonifying the kidney, regulating qi, and promoting blood circulation to resolve stasis, which are consistently applied throughout the therapeutic process.

4.6.1 Internal treatment

Internal treatment should be based on a comprehensive analysis of the duration of disease, pigmentation color, lesion size and location, accompanying symptoms, tongue coating characteristics, and other clinical manifestations. Syndrome differentiation and treatment modification should be guided by the individual patient's presentation.

- Liver Qi stagnation syndrome: Facial pigmentation typically appears bluish-brown, with lesions often presenting in a butterfly-shaped distribution over the cheeks. Patients may experience irritability, emotional depression, menstrual irregularities, a red tongue, and a wiry pulse. The treatment principle focuses on soothing the liver, relieving emotional constraint, and regulating qi and blood. The commonly used decoction is a modified Xiaoyao San, and proprietary Chinese medicines include Xiaoyao Wan, Jiawei Xiaoyao Wan, Shugan San, and Chaihu Shugan San.

- Qi stagnation with blood stasis syndrome: Skin lesions usually appear yellowish-brown, accompanied by irritability, distending pain in the chest and hypochondria, a dark tongue, thin white coating, and a deep, thready pulse. Treatment aims to soothe the liver, regulate Qi, remove blood stasis, and dredge the meridians. The representative prescription is a modified Taohong Siwu Tang, and the commonly used proprietary medicine is Xuefu Zhuyu Oral Liquid.

- Spleen deficiency with damp obstruction syndrome: Lesions are often light brown or gray-brown, mainly distributed around the mouth. Patients may have sallow complexion, fatigue, shortness of breath, reluctance to speak, loose stools, abdominal distension, a pale tongue with thin and slightly greasy coating, and a soft, thready, and moderate pulse. The treatment strategy includes strengthening the spleen, regulating qi, eliminating dampness, and unblocking the meridians. The typical decoction is a modified Shenling Baizhu San, which is also available as a commonly used patent medicine.

- Liver and kidney Yin deficiency syndrome: Pigmentation is typically dark brown, often accompanied by soreness and weakness in the lumbar region and knees, dizziness, tinnitus, dry eyes, menstrual irregularities, tidal fever, red tongue with little coating, and a deep, thready pulse. The therapeutic approach involves nourishing and tonifying the liver and kidney. A modified Liuwei Dihuang Wan is commonly prescribed, and Liuwei Dihuang Wan is also widely used in proprietary form.

4.6.2 External therapies in traditional Chinese medicine

In clinical practice, traditional Chinese medicine (TCM) is often applied externally in the form of powdered herbal preparations made into creams, facial masks, or alginate masks. Additionally, the residue from decocted internal prescriptions may be used for fumigation followed by wet application. Commonly used topical herbs include *Bletilla striata* (Baiji), *Typhonium giganteum* (Baifuzi), *Bombyx batryticatus* (Baijiangcan), pearl powder, *Angelica sinensis* (Danggui), *Ligusticum chuanxiong* (Chuanxiong), *Leonurus japonicus* (Yimucao), *Ampelopsis japonica* (Bailian), *Trichosanthes kirilowii* (Tianhuafen), *Poria cocos* (Baifuling), *Coix lacryma-jobi* (Yiyiren), *Schizonepeta tenuifolia* (Jingjie), *Benincasa hispida* (Dongguaren), *Prunus armeniaca* (Xingren), and *Centella asiatica* (Jixuecao). The typical duration of external TCM therapy ranges from 2 to 6 months.

In summary, with the ongoing advances in the understanding of melasma pathogenesis and improvements in clinical diagnostic and therapeutic techniques, treatment outcomes have significantly improved in recent years. Given the limited efficacy of monotherapy, it is essential to avoid triggering factors and incorporate photoprotection throughout the entire course of treatment. Individualized and comprehensive treatment strategies should be formulated based on clinical staging and classification, taking into account pigmentation, inflammation, vascular involvement, skin barrier integrity, and photoaging.

5. Future directions and research opportunities

5.1 Long-term management challenges

The long-term management of melasma is hindered by two key challenges: suboptimal patient adherence and the chronic, recurrent nature of the disease. Although melasma is more prevalent among individuals with darker skin tones, adherence to sun protection has been found to be low. For instance, only 7.6% of patients have been reported to reapply sunscreen at two-hour intervals, as recommended by clinical guidelines [12]. Effective long-term management requires more than sunscreen use alone. Due to the multifactorial etiology of melasma, combination therapy involving multiple agents is often necessary. However, this approach increases the risk of adverse reactions, such as contact dermatitis and allergic responses. In addition, the psychosocial burden of melasma has yet to be incorporated into clinical treatment frameworks. Some patients experience persistent low self-esteem and impaired quality of life even after clinical improvement, underscoring the need for psychosocial support as part of comprehensive disease management [75].

5.2 Challenges in broad-spectrum light photoprotection

Melasma relapse is also strongly associated with exposure to visible light besides UV, particularly blue light. While conventional sunscreens primarily block UVA and UVB rays, effective blue light protection requires the use of physical barriers, which are often cosmetically unappealing and poorly tolerated. Consequently, there is an urgent need for the development of broad-spectrum sunscreens and an expanded range of physical sunscreen shades to improve both adherence and clinical efficacy [13, 75].

5.3 Investigation of polyamine metabolism pathways

Recent studies have shown that the expression of ornithine decarboxylase 1 (ODC1), the rate-limiting enzyme in polyamine synthesis, is significantly upregulated in melanocytes from hyperpigmented melasma lesions. However, the molecular mechanisms by which polyamines influence tyrosinase (TYR) activity—potentially *via* oxidative stress intermediates such as hydrogen peroxide (H_2O_2)—remain inadequately elucidated. Future research could focus on elucidating the specific roles of the two primary polyamine degradation pathways—spermine oxidase (SMOX) and spermidine/spermine-N1-acetyltransferase (SAT1)—by applying shRNA techniques to determine their relative contributions to melanin production. As polyamine homeostasis is tightly regulated at the cellular level through synthesis, degradation, and transport, targeting this pathway may inadvertently affect other physiological functions, including cellular proliferation and immune response, thus complicating drug development. For example, the polyamine degradation inhibitor MDL72527 has been shown to inhibit putrescine-induced pigmentation, but its systemic effects remain unclear [76].

5.4 The application of AI

Artificial intelligence is increasingly employed in the differential diagnosis of inflammatory and infectious skin disorders. Melasma, as a common pigmentary condition, may also benefit from AI-assisted diagnostic tools. One study developed an AI-based diagnostic model utilizing the five imaging modes of the VISIA system. Among single-mode inputs, the "BROWN SPOTS" mode achieved the highest performance (accuracy: 94.42%; AUC: 98.57%). Multi-modal fusion of "NORMAL + BROWN SPOTS + UV SPOTS" further improved accuracy to 97.4% and AUC to 99.28%, underscoring the utility of integrated imaging modalities. These technologies provide a fast and objective diagnostic option, particularly valuable for primary care settings and remote areas [77].

Additionally, a portable spectral-domain optical coherence tomography (SD-OCT) system has been developed to obtain high-resolution, three-dimensional

DOI: http://dx.doi.org/10.5772/intechopen.1012673

skin images. Utilizing deep learning algorithms, the system achieved 94.2% diagnostic accuracy in distinguishing healthy skin, melasma, and surrounding tissue. Notably, the device can visualize structural changes in both the epidermis and dermis, such as basement membrane damage and microvascular proliferation, which are characteristic of melasma [78].

Despite these advances, current AI technologies are not yet suitable for widespread clinical application. Key limitations include the use of small training datasets and the underrepresentation of diverse Fitzpatrick skin types, potentially compromising diagnostic accuracy in populations disproportionately affected by melasma. Furthermore, demographic and clinical metadata have not been sufficiently integrated into existing AI models, and standardized approaches for quantifying disease severity remain undeveloped. Future efforts should be directed toward the curation of more diverse datasets and the development of robust, generalizable algorithms to improve diagnostic accuracy and enhance clinical applicability [77, 79].

6. Conclusions

In conclusion, although melasma has a high prevalence and a complex pathogenesis, advances in noninvasive skin diagnostic technologies, particularly dermoscopy and RCM, have enabled more accurate diagnosis of the condition. Building upon conventional treatment approaches, novel techniques such as microneedle injection and nanoparticle-based therapies are increasingly being applied, while AI is further enhancing the development of personalized treatment strategies. This chapter provides a comprehensive overview of current evidence and emerging trends in melasma diagnosis and therapy, serving as a clinical guide for dermatologists and researchers.

Author contributions

All authors contributed to the study conception and design. LZ is responsible for article writing, illustration drawing, and manuscript preparation. BW, YZ, XY, ZC, SS, and QZ participated in reviewing and revising the manuscript. XW and PW critically revised the work, and they contributed equally to this work and should be considered co-corresponding authors. All authors read and approved the final manuscript.

Conflict of interest

The authors declare no conflict of interest.

Author details

Liyuan Zhou, Bingyu Wang, Yiting Zhao, Xidie Yin, Zhi Cao, Shuzhan Shen, Xiuli Wang, Qingyu Zeng and Peiru Wang*
Institute of Photomedicine, Shanghai Skin Disease Hospital, School of Medicine, Tongji University, Shanghai, China

*Address all correspondence to: wangpeiru@tongji.edu.cn

References

[1] Ortonne JP, Arellano I, Berneburg M, Cestari T, Chan H, Grimes P, et al. A global survey of the role of ultraviolet radiation and hormonal influences in the development of melasma. Journal of the European Academy of Dermatology and Venereology. 2009;**23**(11):1254-1262

[2] Kwon SH, Hwang YJ, Lee SK, Park KC. Heterogeneous pathology of melasma and its clinical implications. International Journal of Molecular Sciences. 2016;**17**(6):5110

[3] Rajanala S, Maymone MBC, Vashi NA. Melasma pathogenesis: A review of the latest research, pathological findings, and investigational therapies. Dermatology Online Journal. 2019;**25**(10):13030

[4] He L, Xu A, Gao T, Lei T, et al. Consensus on diagnosis and treatment of melasma in China (2021 version). Chinese Journal of Dermatology. 2021;**54**(2):110-115

[5] Balkrishnan R, McMichael AJ, Camacho FT, Saltzberg F, Housman TS, Grummer S, et al. Development and validation of a health-related quality of life instrument for women with melasma. The British Journal of Dermatology. 2003;**149**(3):572-577

[6] Cestari TF, Hexsel D, Viegas ML, Azulay L, Hassun K, Almeida AR, et al. Validation of a melasma quality of life questionnaire for Brazilian Portuguese language: The MelasQoL-BP study and improvement of QoL of melasma patients after triple combination therapy. The British Journal of Dermatology. 2006;**156**(Suppl. 1):13-20

[7] Dominguez AR, Balkrishnan R, Ellzey AR, Pandya AG. Melasma in Latina patients: Cross-cultural adaptation and validation of a quality-of-life questionnaire in Spanish language. Journal of the American Academy of Dermatology. 2006;**55**(1):59-66

[8] Freitag FM, Cestari TF, Leopoldo LR, Paludo P, Boza JC. Effect of melasma on quality of life in a sample of women living in southern Brazil. Journal of the European Academy of Dermatology and Venereology. 2008;**22**(6):655-662

[9] Chen Y, Vellaichamy G, Schneider SL, Kong W, Liu Z. Exposure factors in the occurrence and development of melasma (review). Experimental and Therapeutic Medicine. 2024;**27**(4):131

[10] Sofía Bernarda Ortiz Á, Johanna Paola Gaibor B, Claudia Gabriela Jara M, Diana Marisol Berrezueta R, De Los M, Ángeles Arévalo G, et al. Melasma etiology and treatment: A systematic review. EPRA International Journal of Multidisciplinary Research (IJMR). 2024;**10**(1):276-280

[11] Esposito ACC, Cassiano DP, da Silva CN, Lima PB, Dias JAF, Hassun K, et al. Update on melasma-part I: Pathogenesis. Dermatology and Therapy (Heidelberg). 2022;**12**(9):1967-1988

[12] Morgado-Carrasco D, Piquero-Casals J, Granger C, Trullàs C, Passeron T. Melasma: The need for tailored photoprotection to improve clinical outcomes. Photodermatology, Photoimmunology & Photomedicine. 2022;**38**(6):515-521

[13] Regazzetti C, Sormani L, Debayle D, Bernerd F, Tulic MK, De Donatis GM, et al. Melanocytes sense blue light and regulate pigmentation through Opsin-3. The Journal of Investigative Dermatology. 2018;**138**(1):171-178

[14] Kim NH, Cheong KA, Lee TR, Lee AY. PDZK1 upregulation in estrogen-related hyperpigmentation in melasma. The Journal of Investigative Dermatology. 2012;**132**(11):2622-2631

[15] Park TJ, Kim M, Kim H, Park SY, Park KC, Ortonne JP, et al. Wnt inhibitory factor (WIF)-1 promotes melanogenesis in normal human melanocytes. Pigment Cell & Melanoma Research. 2014;**27**(1):72-81

[16] Kim JY, Lee TR, Lee AY. Reduced WIF-1 expression stimulates skin hyperpigmentation in patients with melasma. The Journal of Investigative Dermatology. 2013;**133**(1):191-200

[17] Zhu JW, Ni YJ, Tong XY, Guo X, Wu XP, Lu ZF. Tranexamic acid inhibits angiogenesis and melanogenesis in vitro by targeting VEGF receptors. International Journal of Medical Sciences. 2020;**17**(7):903-911

[18] Masub N, Nguyen JK, Austin E, Jagdeo J. The vascular component of melasma: A systematic review of laboratory, diagnostic, and therapeutic evidence. Dermatologic Surgery. 2020;**46**(12):1642-1650

[19] Hakozaki T, Wang J, Laughlin T, Jarrold B, Zhao W, Furue M. Role of interleukin-6 and endothelin-1 receptors in enhanced melanocyte dendricity of facial spots and suppression of their ligands by niacinamide and tranexamic acid. Journal of the European Academy of Dermatology and Venereology. 2024;**38**(Suppl. 2):3-10

[20] Espósito ACC, Cassiano DP, Bagatin E, Miot HA. Regarding the alterations in oxidative stress status induced by melasma treatments. Archives of Dermatological Research. 2021;**313**(8):705-706

[21] Platsidaki E, Markantoni V, Nicolaidou E, Katoulis A, Rigopoulos D, Stratigos AJ, et al. Melasma: A clinical and epidemiological single-group observational study in the Greek population. Dermatology and Therapy (Heidelberg). 2024;**14**(11):3183-3192

[22] KrupaShankar DS, Somani VK, Kohli M, Sharad J, Ganjoo A, Kandhari S, et al. A cross-sectional, multicentric clinico-epidemiological study of melasma in India. Dermatology and Therapy (Heidelberg). 2014;**4**(1):71-81

[23] Neagu N, Conforti C, Agozzino M, Marangi GF, Morariu SH, Pellacani G, et al. Melasma treatment: A systematic review. The Journal of Dermatological Treatment. 2022;**33**(4):1816-1837

[24] Majid I, Aleem S. Melasma: Update on epidemiology, clinical presentation, assessment, and scoring. Journal of Skin and Stem Cell. 2022;**8**(4):e120283

[25] Chatterjee M, Neema S. Dermoscopy of pigmentary disorders in brown skin. Dermatologic Clinics. 2018;**36**(4):473-485

[26] Punchihewa N, Rodrigues M. A comprehensive review of dermoscopy in melasma. Clinical and Experimental Dermatology. 2024;**49**(9):956-960

[27] Navya A, Pai V. Comparison of dermoscope and woods lamp as a tool to study melanin depth in melasma. Indian Dermatology Online Journal. 2022;**13**(3):366-369

[28] Bala HR, Lee S, Wong C, Pandya AG, Rodrigues M. Oral tranexamic acid for the treatment of melasma: A review. Dermatologic Surgery. 2018;**44**(6):814-825

[29] Farabi B, Khan S, Jamgochian M, Atak MF, Jain M, Rao BK. The role of reflectance confocal microscopy in the diagnosis and management

of pigmentary disorders: A review. Journal of Cosmetic Dermatology. 2023;**22**(12):3213-3222

[30] Duman N, Yaman B, Oraloğlu G, Karaarslan I. The use of in vivo reflectance confocal microscopy for the diagnosis and classification of melasma. Indian Journal of Dermatology. 2023;**68**(6):666-668

[31] Harumi O, Goh CL. The effect of melasma on the quality of life in a sample of women living in Singapore. The Journal of Clinical and Aesthetic Dermatology. 2016;**9**(1):21-24

[32] Shin JA, Sun M, Jeong JM. Borage oil treated with immobilized lipase inhibits melanogenesis. Lipids. 2020;**55**(6):649-659

[33] Lu Q, Yang C, Wu J, Wei Z, Xu S, Wang C, et al. Confocal laser scanning microscopy, a diagnostic alternative for five pigmented lesions on the face: An observational study. Skin Research and Technology. 2019;**25**(6):871-876

[34] Calacattawi R, Alshahrani M, Aleid M, Aleid F, Basamih K, Alsugair G, et al. Tranexamic acid as a therapeutic option for melasma management: Meta-analysis and systematic review of randomized controlled trials. The Journal of Dermatological Treatment. 2024;**35**(1):2361106

[35] Kwon HJ, Suh JH, Ko EJ, Kim BJ. Combination treatment of propranolol, minocycline, and tranexamic acid for effective control of rosacea. Dermatologic Therapy. 2017;**30**(3):e12439

[36] Forbat E, Al-Niaimi F, Ali FR. The emerging importance of tranexamic acid in dermatology. Clinical and Experimental Dermatology. 2020;**45**(4):445-449

[37] Fioranelli M, Jafferany M, Wollina U, Tirant M, Van Thuong N, Lotti T. New local treatments for different types of melasma: Vascular type vs nonvascular type. A randomized polycentric study. Dermatologic Therapy. 2020;**33**(3):e13300

[38] Banihashemi M, Zabolinejad N, Jaafari MR, Salehi M, Jabari A. Comparison of therapeutic effects of liposomal tranexamic acid and conventional hydroquinone on melasma. Journal of Cosmetic Dermatology. 2015;**14**(3):174-177

[39] Pazyar N, Yaghoobi R, Zeynalie M, Vala S. Comparison of the efficacy of intradermal injected tranexamic acid vs hydroquinone cream in the treatment of melasma. Clinical, Cosmetic and Investigational Dermatology. 2019;**12**:115-122

[40] Chen LY, Kang YN, Hoang KD, Chen KH, Chen C. Intradermal injection of tranexamic acid for the treatment of adult melasma: A systematic review and meta-analysis of randomized controlled trials. Facial Plastic Surgery & Aesthetic Medicine. 2025;**27**(4):305-312

[41] Demirbas A, Ulutas Demirbas G, Diremsizoglu E, Esen M. Dual benefits of oral tranexamic acid: Reducing melasma severity and inflammation. Journal of Cosmetic Dermatology. 2025;**24**(5):e70257

[42] Chen XY, Chen Y, Qu CJ, Pan ZH, Qin Y, Zhang X, et al. Vitamin C induces human melanoma A375 cell apoptosis via Bax- and Bcl-2-mediated mitochondrial pathways. Oncology Letters. 2019;**18**(4):3880-3886

[43] Carr AC, Maggini S. Vitamin C and immune function. Nutrients. 2017;**9**:11

[44] Keen MA, Hassan I. Vitamin E in dermatology. Indian Dermatology Online Journal. 2016;**7**(4):311-315

[45] Speeckaert R, Bulat V, Speeckaert MM, van Geel N. The impact of antioxidants on vitiligo and melasma: A scoping review and meta-analysis. Antioxidants (Basel). 2023;**12**(12):2082

[46] Rodrigues M, Pandya AG. Melasma: Clinical diagnosis and management options. The Australasian Journal of Dermatology. 2015;**56**(3):151-163

[47] Sarkar R, Handog EB, Das A, Bansal A, Macarayo MJ, Keshavmurthy V, et al. Topical and systemic therapies in melasma: A systematic review. Indian Dermatology Online Journal. 2023;**14**(6):769-781

[48] González-Molina V, Martí-Pineda A, González N. Topical treatments for melasma and their mechanism of action. The Journal of Clinical and Aesthetic Dermatology. 2022;**15**(5):19-28

[49] Tekam PS, Belgaumkar VA. Combination of autologous platelet rich plasma and hydroquinone 4% is more effective than hydroquinone alone in treatment of melasma: A split-face comparative study. Dermatologic Therapy. 2022;**35**(11):e15761

[50] Boo YC. Arbutin as a skin depigmenting agent with antimelanogenic and antioxidant properties. Antioxidants (Basel). 2021;**10**(7):1129

[51] Tantanasrigul P, Sripha A, Chongmelaxme B. The efficacy of topical cosmetic containing alpha-Arbutin 5% and Kojic acid 2% compared with triple combination cream for the treatment of melasma: A split-face, evaluator-blinded randomized pilot study. Journal of Cosmetic Dermatology. 2025;**24**(1):e16562

[52] Sarkar R, Katoch S. Chemical peels in treatment of melasma. Dermatologic Clinics. 2024;**42**(1):21-32

[53] Agozzino M, Licata G, Giorgio CMR, Babino G, Lupoli A, Sperduti I, et al. Reflectance confocal microscopy assessment of the depigmenting agents complex for melasma treatment. The Journal of Clinical and Aesthetic Dermatology. 2020;**13**(9):41-44

[54] Hoque F, McGrath J, Ebeny SS. Melasma (chloasma): Pathogenesis and treatment. Journal of Biotechnology and Biomedicine. 2022;**05**(04):236-243

[55] Hmingthansanga V, Singh N, Banerjee S, Manickam S, Velayutham R, Natesan S. Improved topical drug delivery: Role of permeation enhancers and advanced approaches. Pharmaceutics. 2022;**14**(12):2818

[56] He X, Jin S, Dai X, Chen L, Xiang L, Zhang C. The emerging role of visible light in melanocyte biology and skin pigmentary disorders: Friend or foe? Journal of Clinical Medicine. 2023;**12**(23):7488

[57] Yi J, Hong T, Zeng H, Li P, Li P, Wang S, et al. A meta-analysis-based assessment of intense pulsed light for treatment of melasma. Aesthetic Plastic Surgery. 2020;**44**(3):947-952

[58] Hassan AM, Elfar NN, Rizk OM, Eissa NY. Pulsed dye laser versus intense pulsed light in melasma: A split-face comparative study. The Journal of Dermatological Treatment. 2018;**29**(7):725-732

[59] Kong SH, Suh HS, Choi YS. Treatment of melasma with pulsed-dye laser and 1,064-nm Q-switched Nd:YAG laser: A split-face study. Annals of Dermatology. 2018;**30**(1):1-7

[60] Xu J, Pu Y. Q-switched laser combined with intense pulsed laser in the treatment of melasma based on reflection confocal microscope. Computational

and Mathematical Methods in Medicine. 2022;**2022**:4413130

[61] Piccolo D, Fusco I, Crisman G, Zingoni T, Conforti C. Efficacy and safety of Q-switched 1064/532 nm Nd:YAG lasers on benign hypermelanosis in dark-skinned individuals-A preliminary study. Journal of Clinical Medicine. 2024;**13**(6):1615

[62] Lee YS, Lee YJ, Lee JM, Han TY, Lee JH, Choi JE. The low-fluence Q-switched Nd:YAG laser treatment for melasma: A systematic review. Medicina (Kaunas, Lithuania). 2022;**58**(7):936

[63] Lee MC, Lin YF, Hu S, Huang YL, Chang SL, Cheng CY, et al. A split-face study: Comparison of picosecond alexandrite laser and Q-switched Nd:YAG laser in the treatment of melasma in Asians. Lasers in Medical Science. 2018;**33**(8):1733-1738

[64] Huth S, Marquardt Y, Huth L, Gerber PA, Baron JM. Molecular insights into the effects of laser-induced optical breakdown (LIOB) after 1064 nm picosecond laser irradiation using a novel melanocyte-containing 3D skin model. Lasers in Medical Science. 2025;**40**(1):223

[65] Waibel JS, Schallen KP. Non-ablative fractional 1940-nm diode laser for skin resurfacing and treatment of benign pigmented lesions. Lasers in Surgery and Medicine. 2025;**57**(1):63-70

[66] Feng J, Shen S, Song X, Xiang W. Efficacy and safety of laser-assisted delivery of tranexamic acid for the treatment of melasma: A systematic review and meta-analysis. Journal of Cosmetic and Laser Therapy. 2022;**24**(6-8):73-79

[67] Mekawy KMM, Sadek A, Seddeik Abdel-Hameed AK. Micro-needling versus fractional carbon dioxide laser for delivery of tranexamic acid in the treatment of melasma: A split-face study. Journal of Cosmetic Dermatology. 2021;**20**(2):460-465

[68] Acar A, Ozturk A, Sokmen N, Unal I, Ertam SI. Evaluation of platelet-rich plasma efficacy in melasma. Journal of Cosmetic and Laser Therapy. 2022;**24**(1-5):36-39

[69] Jiryis B, Toledano O, Avitan-Hersh E, Khamaysi Z. Management of melasma: Laser and other therapies-review study. Journal of Clinical Medicine. 2024;**13**(5):1468

[70] Abd Elraouf IG, Obaid ZM, Fouda I. Intradermal injection of tranexamic acid versus platelet-rich plasma in the treatment of melasma: A split-face comparative study. Archives of Dermatological Research. 2023;**315**(6):1763-1770

[71] Chen W, Jian X, Yu B. Review of applications of microneedling in melasma. Journal of Cosmetic Dermatology. 2025;**24**(1):e16707

[72] Bailey AJM, Li HO, Tan MG, Cheng W, Dover JS. Microneedling as an adjuvant to topical therapies for melasma: A systematic review and meta-analysis. Journal of the American Academy of Dermatology. 2022;**86**(4):797-810

[73] Simin H, Siliang X, Wei C, Ping D, Erlong L, Jianbo Z. Efficacy of microneedle as an assisted therapy for melasma: A meta-analysis and systematic review of randomized controlled trials. Aesthetic Plastic Surgery. 2025;**49**(6):1755-1769

[74] Hofny ERM, Younis AH, Badary DM, Elnaggar MG, Eleraky NE, Abdel-Bary IM, et al. Comparative study

of different treatment modalities for melasma: Introducing a novel nanotechnology-based tranexamic acid microemulsion. Archives of Dermatological Research. 2025;**317**(1):792

[75] Liu W, Chen Q, Xia Y. New mechanistic insights of melasma. Clinical, Cosmetic and Investigational Dermatology. 2023;**16**:429-442

[76] Sridharan A, Shi M, Leo VI, Subramaniam N, Lim TC, Uemura T, et al. The polyamine putrescine promotes human epidermal melanogenesis. The Journal of Investigative Dermatology. 2020;**140**(10):2032-40.e1

[77] Liu L, Liang C, Xue Y, Chen T, Chen Y, Lan Y, et al. An intelligent diagnostic model for melasma based on deep learning and multimode image input. Dermatology and Therapy (Heidelberg). 2023;**13**(2):569-579

[78] Cao X, Lu Y, Zhu T, Yan Z, Li K, Mo J. Diagnosis and post-treatment follow-up evaluation of melasma using optical coherence tomography and deep learning. Journal of Biophotonics. 2025;**18**(6):e70006

[79] Escalé-Besa A, Vidal-Alaball J, Miró Catalina Q, Gracia VHG, Marin-Gomez FX, Fuster-Casanovas A. The use of artificial intelligence for skin disease diagnosis in primary care settings: A systematic review. Healthcare (Basel). 2024;**12**(12):1192

Chapter 3

Epigenetics of Solar Lentigines: Molecular Insights into Photoaging and Skin Pigmentation Disorders

Nomakhosi Mpofana, Mokgadi Ursula Makgobole and Pavitra Pillay

Abstract

Chronic exposure to the sun can significantly impact the skin, often resulting in solar lentigines (SL), also known as age spots. These marks are clear signs of photoaging and hyperpigmentation, particularly in those with fair skin. While traditionally linked to extended ultraviolet (UV) exposure and increased melanocyte activity, SLs are now recognized as involving more profound molecular disruptions. Epigenetic processes play a crucial role in this, modifying gene expression without altering the underlying DNA sequence. These epigenetic changes leave lasting effects on skin cells, promoting processes such as melanogenesis, cellular aging, and chronic inflammation. The interaction of these pathways leads to persistent pigmentation and structural changes in the skin that define SL. For instance, cellular aging contributes to the skin's aged appearance through the senescence-associated secretory phenotype (SASP), which encourages local inflammation and melanin production. At the same time, melanocyte regulation is disrupted due to epigenetically driven gene control issues, causing uneven pigment distribution. New therapeutic approaches are focusing on these underlying epigenetic factors. Sirtuins, a group of proteins involved in DNA repair and metabolic regulation, along with specific microRNAs that influence pigmentation and inflammatory signaling, are being explored for their potential to reverse or lessen SL development. These treatments aim not only to address visible skin changes but also to restore cellular balance. Understanding the epigenetic basis of solar lentigines connects dermatological symptoms with molecular pathology. This comprehensive review emphasizes the importance of early detection and targeted treatment while also highlighting the need for interdisciplinary strategies in managing solar lentigines and skin aging.

Keywords: solar lentigines, ultraviolet radiation, photoaging, epigenetic regulation, DNA methylation

1. Introduction

The skin, as the largest and most visible organ of the human body, functions as a vital barrier against numerous environmental threats, with solar radiation being a primary concern [1, 2]. According to Dorosz and colleagues [3], over time, exposure to ultraviolet (UV) rays and the intrinsic aging process induce changes in the skin. Among the most prevalent and noticeable of these changes is the appearance of solar lentigines, informally referred to as "age spots" or "liver spots" [3, 4]. These benign hyperpigmented lesions typically manifest on sun-exposed areas of the body, such as the face, chest, arms, and dorsal surfaces of the hands [5]. They vary in hue from light to dark brown and display a range of sizes. With advancing age, the incidence of these lesions increases, serving as a visible testament to cumulative sun exposure [6]. Solar lentigines are exceedingly common, affecting over 90% of individuals with fair skin who are above the age of 60 [7, 8]. For many individuals, these lesions represent a cosmetic concern, thereby fueling a substantial market for therapeutic interventions [9]. More critically, they signify extensive sun exposure, which is the primary etiological factor for all forms of skin cancer [10]. Although solar lentigines themselves infrequently undergo malignant transformation, they may occasionally mimic more serious dermatological conditions [1], underscoring the necessity for thorough medical assessment. According to Tumsutti and Rojhirunsakool [11], the pathogenesis of solar lentigines has been attributed largely to the impact of solar radiation on cutaneous cells. This perspective posits that prolonged UV exposure leads to either an increase in the number or activity of melanocytes, the pigment-producing cells, resulting in hyperpigmentation [12]. At the molecular level, this process involves UV-induced DNA damage, the generation of reactive oxygen species, and the release of various factors that further stimulate melanocyte activity [12, 13].

However, this conventional understanding does not fully explain the variability in susceptibility to these lesions among individuals or their persistence over time [13, 14]. Recent advancements in the field of epigenetics have begun to provide novel insights. Epigenetics examines how gene expression can be modulated without changes to the DNA sequence itself, through mechanisms such as DNA methylation [15] and histone modifications [16]. These epigenetic modifications, influenced by environmental factors like sun exposure, play significant roles in skin aging, inflammation, and oncogenesis [14, 17, 18]. This chapter aims to provide a comprehensive examination of solar lentigines, integrating clinical observations with traditional etiological theories and the growing significance of epigenetics. Exploring how these epigenetic modifications are increasingly recognized as key in the development and characteristics of solar lentigines potentially paves the way for innovative preventive and therapeutic strategies for this common manifestation of photodamaged skin.

Figure 1 offers a brief visual representation of extrinsic skin aging, showing how environmental and lifestyle factors accelerate the decline of skin health. It compares the well-organized, robust structure of youthful skin, marked by plentiful, undamaged collagen and elastin and uniformly spread melanin, with the deteriorated condition of older skin. The illustration reveals that prolonged exposure to factors such as UV radiation, air pollution, stress, and smoking results in widespread cellular aging. This leads to fragmented collagen and elastin, excessive production and clustering of melanin by aging melanocytes (resulting in hyperpigmentation), and the emission of inflammatory signals (SASP) by aging fibroblasts, perpetuating a cycle of damage and visible aging [19].

Figure 2 below illustrates the evolutionary path and geographical spread of diversity in human skin color. It emphasizes how differences in skin tone have developed over time as adaptations to varying levels of ultraviolet (UV) radiation in different parts of the world. Darker skin tones primarily evolved in populations near the equator to shield against intense UV exposure, while lighter skin tones emerged in groups that

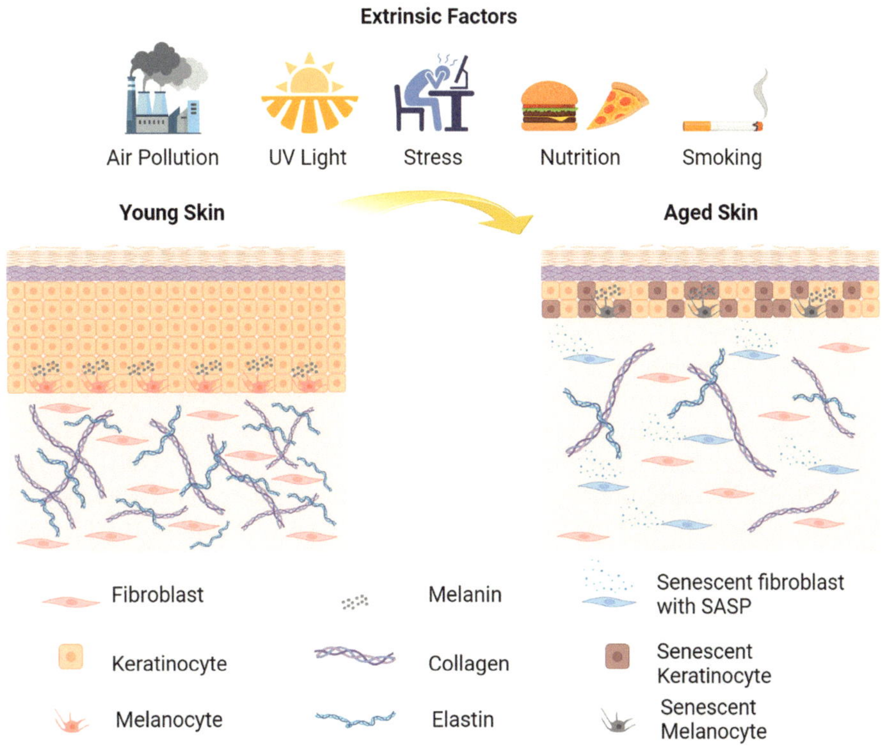

Figure 1.
Visual representation of extrinsic skin aging, showing how environmental and lifestyle factors accelerate the decline of skin health [19].

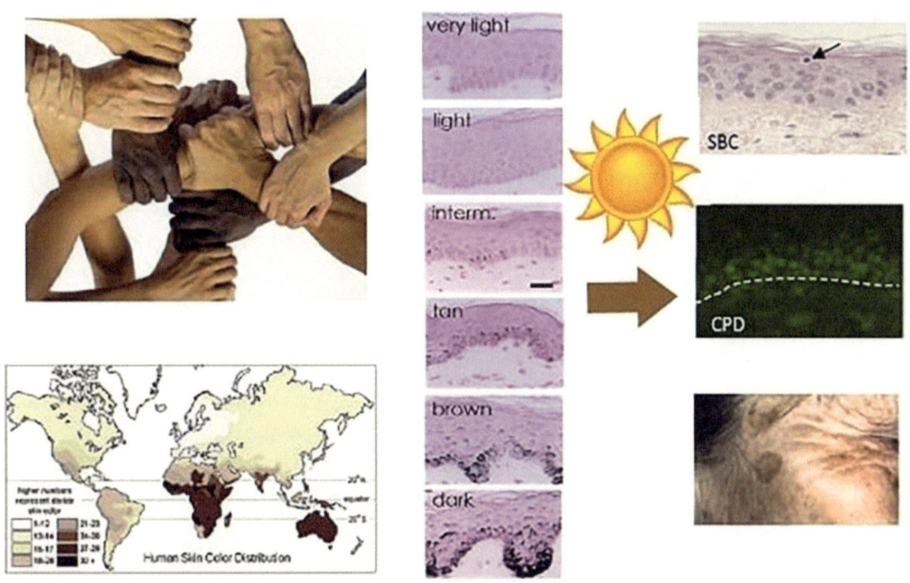

Figure 2.
Skin pigmentation diversity- evolution of skin pigmentation diversity [20].

migrated to higher latitudes with reduced UV radiation, facilitating vitamin D production [20, 21]. The figure highlights the intricate relationship between genetic, environmental, and evolutionary influences that shape the global range of skin pigmentation.

2. Solar lentigines and photoaging

Solar lentigines (SL), commonly known as age spots or liver spots, are indicative of photoaged skin [22]. These lesions present as hyperpigmented macules mainly on sun-exposed regions such as the face, forearms, and hands [23]. According to Hasegawa, Fujiwara [23] SL are among the earliest noticeable indicators of photoaging and may emerge as early as the third decade of life, particularly in individuals with frequent sun exposure. Histologically, SL demonstrate several structural changes, including enhanced vascularization, which is characterized by increased blood flow, vessel density, and elevated expression of vascular endothelial growth factor (VEGF) [24]. Additionally, there is a significant increase in macrophage infiltration in the affected skin, indicating an inflammatory component [25]. Genetic predisposition also contributes to this condition; specific variants in the telomerase reverse transcriptase (TERT) gene have been linked to an increased susceptibility to SL, highlighting the multifactorial etiology that involves both environmental and genetic factors [26].

Figure 3 illustrates a series of four images that serve as a striking visual case study, documenting the progression of a solar lentigo over 5 years using two sophisticated imaging techniques. The top row (a, b) displays dermoscopic images, highlighting the macroscopic changes: the lesion becomes noticeably darker and more prominent as time passes. The bottom row (c, d) provides a more detailed, cellular-level perspective through reflectance confocal microscopy (RCM). The initial RCM image (c) reveals the typical organized, ring-like "cobblestone" pattern of pigmented cells at the dermal-epidermal junction. After 5 years (d), this distinct structure has deteriorated into a chaotic and irregular pattern. Collectively, these images compellingly demonstrate that solar lentigines are not static marks but are dynamically evolving, with their visible darkening reflecting a significant disorganization of the underlying cellular architecture [27].

Photoaging is characterized by the premature aging of the skin resulting from prolonged exposure to ultraviolet (UV) radiation [28]. At the cellular and molecular levels, photoaging is distinguished by two principal pathways of damage: direct UV-induced damage to DNA and other macromolecules and indirect oxidative damage mediated by the generation of reactive oxygen species (ROS) [28, 29]. These mechanisms culminate in inflammation, degradation of extracellular matrix proteins (notably collagen and elastin), apoptosis, mitochondrial dysfunction, and immune dysregulation [29]. Immune system remodeling is a prominent characteristic of photoaging. Prolonged exposure to ultraviolet (UV) radiation results in both localized and systemic immunosuppression, which is marked by an increase in regulatory immune cells [30] and manifestations of immunosenescence patterns that resemble those observed in natural aging [31]. This impaired immune surveillance may intensify pigmentary alterations and inflammation. Autophagy, a cellular mechanism essential to recycling and protection, has been recognized as a potential modulator of photoaging [29, 31]. While autophagy aids in the removal of damaged cellular components and mitigates damage associated with reactive oxygen species (ROS), its precise role in the prevention or reversal of photoaging remains an area of active research [31].

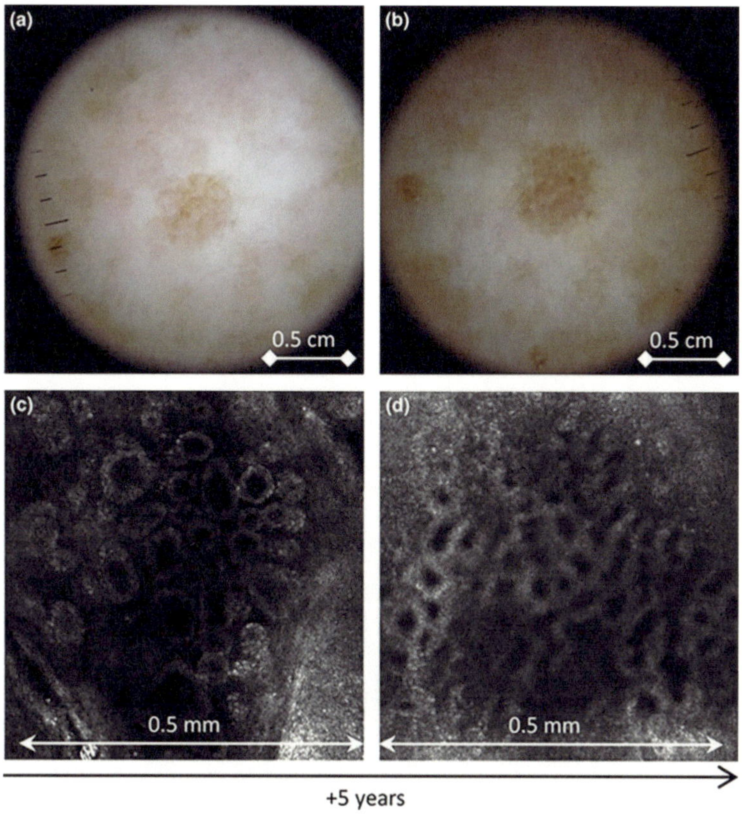

Figure 3.
Illustration of a dermoscopy picture (A, B) and a confocal image at dermal-epidermal level (C, D) at the first evaluation (A, C) and 5 years later (B, D), showing progressive deformation and compression of the dermal papillary rings [27].

3. Environmental triggers: UV radiation and oxidative stress

The primary environmental driver of both SL and photoaging is chronic UV radiation, particularly UVA and UVB wavelengths [32]. These rays penetrate the skin and generate ROS, leading to DNA mutations, oxidative stress, and long-term structural damage [33]. The cumulative effect of UV exposure disrupts the homeostasis of melanocytes and keratinocytes, contributing to irregular pigmentation and lesion formation [34]. In addition to ultraviolet (UV) radiation, other environmental stressors, such as pollutants and toxicants, have been demonstrated to affect skin aging and pigmentation [34]. Notably, the aryl hydrocarbon receptor (AhR) signaling pathways play a role in the interaction between environmental toxicants and skin cells [33]. This signaling crosstalk contributes to the persistence and exacerbation of pigment spots, such as solar lentigines (SL) [35]. Oxidative stress initiates several intracellular pathways that significantly impact skin health. Notably, the nuclear factor erythroid 2–related factor 2 (NRF2) and nuclear factor kappa-light-chain-enhancer of activated B cells (NF-κB) pathways are of particular importance [36]. Activation of NRF2 enhances antioxidant defenses; however, its dysregulation has been associated with SL formation [37]. Pharmacological targeting of these pathways presents a promising therapeutic strategy for mitigating pigmentation and inflammation linked to photoaging.

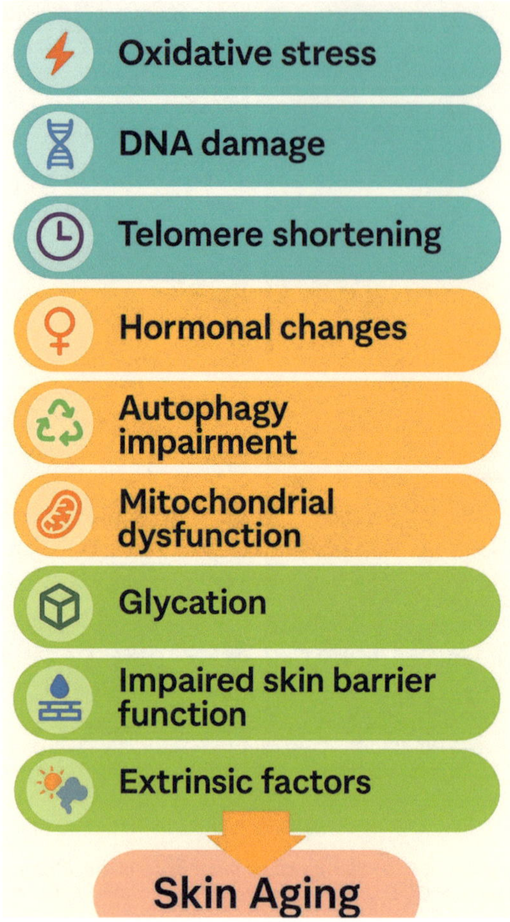

Figure 4.
Diagrammatic illustration of the various factors involved in the process of skin aging [38] [Created with OpenAI, 2025].

Figure 4 presents a schematic summary of the primary biological and environmental elements that play a role in skin aging. This complex process is influenced by both internal and external factors that collectively impact the skin's structure and function over time. As shown, significant factors include oxidative stress, which causes cellular damage, mutations in mitochondrial DNA that disrupt energy metabolism, DNA damage and telomere shortening that hinder cellular replication, hormonal changes that affect skin balance, and reduced autophagy, which diminishes the skin's ability to eliminate damaged components. These interconnected pathways collectively accelerate the visible and functional signs of skin aging.

4. Epigenetic regulation in skin biology

Epigenetics involves heritable modifications in gene expression that do not alter the DNA sequence itself [39]. These modifications function as molecular switches that regulate gene activity in response to environmental, developmental, and physiological signals. In the field of skin biology, epigenetic mechanisms, including DNA methylation, histone modifications, and noncoding RNAs, play a crucial role in maintaining tissue homeostasis, regulating repair processes, and mediating age-associated changes [39, 40]. DNA methylation involves the addition of methyl groups to cytosine bases in CpG islands, typically leading to gene silencing [39]. In the context of skin aging, age-related changes in methylation patterns include global hypomethylation, which can lead to genomic instability, and promoter-specific hypermethylation, which may suppress genes essential for cellular repair and defense [39]. These alterations contribute to the decline in skin structure and function over time [2]. Furthermore, DNA methylation patterns form the basis of the "epigenetic clock," a biomarker that estimates biological age and correlates with both intrinsic and extrinsic aging processes in the skin [41]. Histone modifications, such as acetylation and methylation, are vital for controlling chromatin structure and gene accessibility in skin cells [41]. Acetylation of histones (e.g., H3K9ac, H4K16ac) typically activates gene expression and is associated with youthful, regenerative skin [42], while aging and UV exposure often result in increased histone deacetylase (HDAC) activity, suppressing genes involved in collagen synthesis and antioxidative responses [43]. Conversely, histone methylation presents a more complex regulatory pattern [42]: marks like H3K27me3 are repressive and often accumulate with age, contributing to reduced stem cell renewal and impaired tissue repair, whereas activating marks like H3K4me3 tend to diminish, further limiting the skin's regenerative capacity. Noncoding RNAs, particularly microRNAs (miRNAs) and long noncoding RNAs (lncRNAs), have also emerged as critical epigenetic regulators in skin health [29]. miRNAs such as miR-21, miR-29, and miR-34a modulate processes including keratinocyte proliferation, extracellular matrix remodeling, and cellular senescence [44]. Rorteau, Chevalier [45] states that their dysregulation with age is linked to impaired healing and increased signs of skin aging. lncRNAs like ANCR and TINCR regulate epidermal differentiation and stem cell maintenance, with their altered expression contributing to age-related skin thinning and delayed wound repair [46]. Collectively, these epigenetic mechanisms orchestrate a finely tuned balance of gene expression necessary for skin integrity [47]. Disruptions in this balance, driven by aging or environmental stressors, underlie many structural and functional changes observed in aging skin. Understanding these processes opens new avenues for targeted antiaging therapies and skin rejuvenation strategies.

5. Epigenetic mechanisms in solar lentigines

While the clinical and histological characteristics of solar lentigines have been thoroughly documented, recent studies have highlighted the significant role of epigenetic mechanisms in their pathogenesis [14, 17, 48]. Epigenetic modifications, heritable changes in gene expression that do not involve alterations in the DNA sequence, are crucial in understanding how environmental factors, particularly ultraviolet (UV) radiation, result in persistent pigmentation changes [11].

5.1 UV-induced epigenetic alterations

Ultraviolet (UV) radiation constitutes a significant environmental factor in the pathogenesis of solar lentigines, exerting its effects not only through direct DNA damage but also *via* epigenetic modifications [49]. UV exposure can instigate changes in DNA methylation, histone modifications, and microRNA (miRNA) dysregulation, resulting in aberrant gene expression patterns in keratinocytes and melanocytes. For instance, UVB radiation has been demonstrated to enhance the activity of DNA methyltransferases (DNMTs), leading to hypermethylation of tumor suppressor genes and alterations in the promoters of pigmentation-related genes [50]. Concurrently, UV-induced modifications in histone acetyltransferase (HAT) and deacetylase (HDAC) activity alter histone acetylation levels, thereby affecting chromatin accessibility and the transcription of melanogenic genes [14]. Additionally, miRNAs, which regulate gene expression posttranscriptionally, display altered profiles in UV-exposed skin. Members of the miR-21 and miR-200 families, for example, are involved in inflammation and melanocyte regulation, with their dysregulation contributing to pigmentary disorders, including solar lentigines [32, 51].

5.2 Dysregulation of melanogenesis pathways

Melanogenesis, the process by which melanocytes produce melanin, is meticulously regulated by a complex network of signaling pathways, including the microphthalmia-associated transcription factor (MITF), cAMP/PKA, and Wnt/β-catenin pathways [52]. In the context of solar lentigines, UV-induced epigenetic modifications alter the expression of critical melanogenic regulators [29]. Aberrant promoter methylation or histone modification of MITF or its upstream regulators can lead to sustained activation of melanogenesis even after the cessation of UV exposure [53]. Furthermore, the increased expression of paracrine factors from keratinocytes, such as endothelin-1 and stem cell factor (SCF), can epigenetically enhance melanocyte

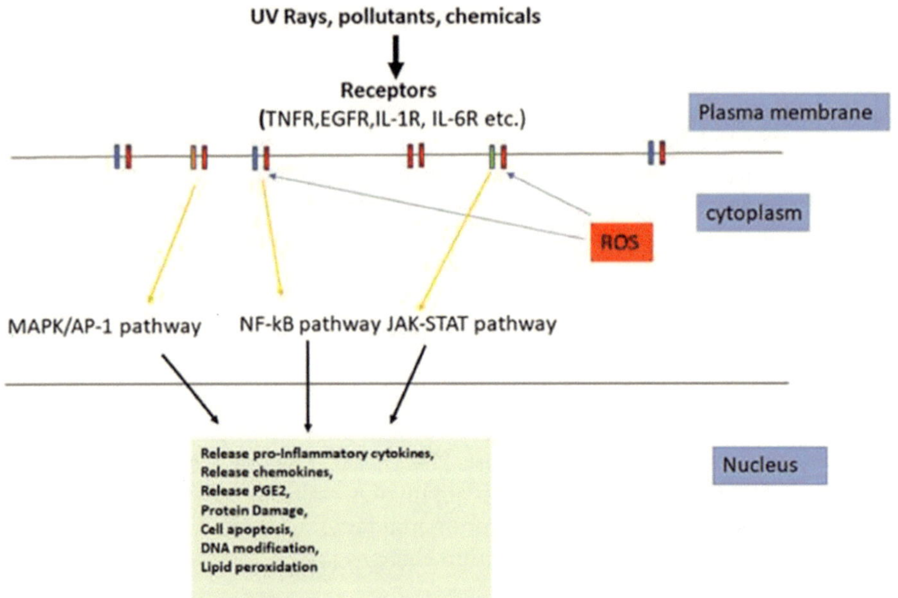

Figure 5.
Illustration of UVR, pollutants, and chemicals that can activate surface receptors either directly or indirectly by activating ROS. Thus, signaling pathways are activated, resulting in protein damage, cell apoptosis, DNA modification, lipid peroxidation, and production of proinflammatory mediators [56]. AP-1: activator protein-1; EGFR: epidermal growth factor receptor; IL-1R: interleukin-1 receptor; IL-6R: interleukin-6 receptor; JAK-STAT: Janus kinase-signal transducer and activator of transcription; MAPK: mitogen-activated protein kinase; NF-κβ: nuclear factor kappa-B; PGE2: Prostaglandin E2. TNFR: tumor necrosis factor receptor; UVR: ultraviolet radiation. The colors yellow, blue, and black arrows indicate direction [56].

activity and melanin synthesis [54]. These alterations result in the focal hyperpigmentation characteristic of solar lentigines [55]. Furthermore, it is observed in many inflammatory disorders that ROS have the most significant effects in MAPK/AP-1, NF-kB, and JAK-STAT signaling pathways (**Figure 5**) [56].

5.3 Senescence and the SASP phenotype

Cellular senescence, characterized by an irreversible cessation of cell proliferation in response to stressors such as ultraviolet radiation, is increasingly acknowledged as a key factor in the development of solar lentigines [57]. In photoaged skin, senescent keratinocytes and fibroblasts accumulate and adopt a senescence-associated secretory phenotype (SASP), which is marked by the secretion of pro-inflammatory cytokines, growth factors, and proteases [58, 59]. The SASP fosters melanocyte hyperactivation and pigment dysregulation by establishing a pro-pigmentary microenvironment [60]. Elements such as interleukin-6 (IL-6), interleukin-8 (IL-8), and matrix metalloproteinases (MMPs) can epigenetically influence the function of adjacent cells through autocrine and paracrine signaling, thereby sustaining a cycle of inflammation and pigmentation [56]. Epigenetically, senescent cells frequently display alterations in chromatin structure, including senescence-associated heterochromatin foci (SAHF) and modified histone marks (e.g., increased H3K9me3), which further promote the SASP phenotype and disrupt tissue homeostasis [61]. **Figure 6** illustrates a schematic representation of skin aging, focusing on the role of cellular senescence.

5.4 Chronic inflammation and pigment imbalance

Chronic low-grade inflammation is a characteristic feature of aging and photo-exposed skin, intricately associated with the development of pigmentary

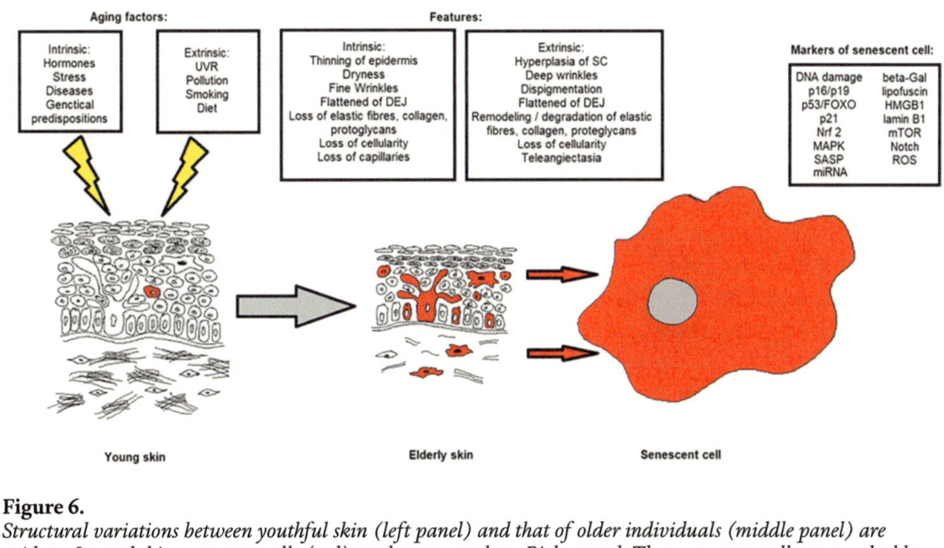

Figure 6.
Structural variations between youthful skin (left panel) and that of older individuals (middle panel) are evident. In aged skin, senescent cells (red) tend to accumulate. Right panel: These senescent cells are marked by increased levels of p21 and p16, the release of the senescence-associated secretory phenotype (SASP), heightened β-galactosidase activity, HMGB1 translocation, decreased laminin B1 expression, buildup of ROS, irregularities in the MAPK-FOXO3, and alterations in the Nrf2, mTOR, and Notch pathways, along with DNA damage. DEJ, dermo-epidermal junction; SC, stratum corneum [59].

disorders such as solar lentigines [25]. Inflammatory mediators not only directly stimulate melanogenesis but also induce epigenetic reprogramming of skin cells. Pro-inflammatory cytokines, including tumor necrosis factor-alpha (TNF-α) and interferon-gamma (IFN-γ), can modulate DNMT and HDAC activity, resulting in the sustained expression of genes involved in inflammation and pigmentation [56, 62]. This epigenetic priming increases the skin's susceptibility to hyperpigmentation upon further environmental insults [29]. Furthermore, the interaction between chronic inflammation and oxidative stress enhances DNA and histone modifications that spread pigment imbalance [52]. Persistent activation of NF-κB signaling, often regulated epigenetically, serves as a critical node linking inflammation, melanocyte stimulation, and the aging process in solar lentigines [54].

6. Molecular crosstalk: Pigmentation, inflammation, and aging

Melanocytes, originating from neural crest cells, play a crucial role in pigmentation through the production of melanin and its subsequent transfer to keratinocytes [63]. As individuals age and in certain inflammatory skin conditions, the function of melanocytes becomes dysregulated [64]. Senescent melanocytes demonstrate impaired melanosome biogenesis, abnormal dendricity, and diminished pigment transfer, resulting in heterogeneous pigmentation patterns such as solar lentigines and post-inflammatory hyperpigmentation (PIH) [60]. Moreover, stress-induced reactive oxygen species (ROS) and DNA damage in melanocytes can initiate premature cellular senescence or apoptosis. This dysfunction not only leads to pigmentary disorders but also contributes to bystander effects, releasing pro-inflammatory cytokines and chemokines that disrupt the homeostasis of surrounding dermal and epidermal tissues [60, 65].

6.1 Inflammatory signaling loops

The interaction between inflammation and pigmentation is complicatedly connected through a feedback loop involving keratinocytes, melanocytes, immune cells, and fibroblasts [66]. Inflammatory cytokines, such as IL-1, IL-6, TNF-α, and IFN-γ, have been demonstrated to affect melanogenesis, by either stimulating or inhibiting melanin production, contingent upon the context and duration of exposure [67]. Chronic low-grade inflammation, a characteristic feature of "inflammaging," disrupts the niche of the basal layer, leading to increased vascular permeability and enhanced leukocyte infiltration [56]. These immune cells secrete matrix metalloproteinases (MMPs) and additional pro-inflammatory mediators, which degrade extracellular matrix (ECM) components and compromise the integrity of the basement membrane. Consequently, this results in increased pigment leakage, uneven melanin deposition, and the perpetuation of the inflammatory loop [39].

6.2 Cellular senescence and structural skin changes

Senescent cells, which accumulate with advancing age, are characterized by irreversible growth arrest, the presence of DNA damage markers such as p16^INK4a and p21^CIP1, and the secretion of the senescence-associated secretory phenotype (SASP) [68, 69]. The SASP comprises pro-inflammatory cytokines, growth factors, and proteases that contribute to extracellular matrix (ECM) degradation, tissue remodeling, and chronic inflammation [69]. In the skin, senescence impacts not only fibroblasts but also melanocytes and keratinocytes [12, 13]. These senescent cells lose their functional capacity and modify their microenvironment, thereby intensifying pigmentary changes and diminishing regenerative ability [3]. The degradation of collagen and elastin by SASP-induced matrix metalloproteinases (MMPs) leads to visible signs of aging, such as wrinkling, loss of elasticity, and uneven pigmentation.

7. Emerging therapeutic approaches

7.1 Epigenetic targets for treatment

Epigenetics encompasses heritable modifications in gene expression that occur without changes to the DNA sequence itself [70]. These modifications, which include DNA methylation, histone modification, and chromatin remodeling, are crucial in regulating cellular identity and function. Aberrant epigenetic changes have been associated with various diseases, notably cancer, neurodegeneration, and autoimmune disorders [71]. Therapeutic strategies targeting the epigenome aim to reverse pathological gene expression profiles. For example, DNA methyltransferase inhibitors (e.g., azacitidine, decitabine) and histone deacetylase inhibitors (e.g., vorinostat, romidepsin) have demonstrated efficacy in hematologic malignancies [8]. Emerging epigenetic therapies now seek enhanced specificity by targeting reader, writer, and eraser proteins that modulate chromatin dynamics. Additionally, CRISPR-based epigenome editing technologies are being investigated for their potential to reprogram gene expression with high precision, offering future prospects for treating both monogenic and complex diseases.

7.2 Role of sirtuins in DNA repair and metabolism

Sirtuins (SIRTs) constitute a family of NAD^+-dependent deacetylases and ADP-ribosyltransferases that integrate cellular energy status with stress responses, DNA repair, and metabolic regulation [72]. Among the seven mammalian sirtuins (SIRT1–SIRT7), several function as nuclear and mitochondrial regulators, playing significant roles in genome maintenance and longevity [73]. For instance, SIRT1 deacetylates p53 and other proteins involved in the DNA damage response, thereby contributing to genomic stability. SIRT6 is essential for base excision repair and telomere maintenance, whereas SIRT3 modulates mitochondrial oxidative stress and energy metabolism [73]. Pharmacological activators of sirtuins, such as resveratrol and novel synthetic compounds, are currently under evaluation for their therapeutic potential in addressing metabolic disorders, cardiovascular disease, neurodegeneration, and aging [74]. Although understanding the context-dependent functions of sirtuins remains challenging, their involvement in both epigenetic regulation and metabolic adaptation positions them as promising targets for multifactorial diseases [75].

7.3 MicroRNAs as therapeutic modulators

MicroRNAs (miRNAs) are small, noncoding RNAs that regulate gene expression post-transcriptionally by binding to complementary sequences on messenger RNAs (mRNAs), resulting in mRNA degradation or inhibition of translation [76]. Dysregulation of miRNAs is implicated in a wide range of diseases, including cancers, cardiovascular diseases, and inflammatory disorders [76, 77]. Therapeutic strategies utilize miRNAs in two primary forms [8, 30]: miRNA mimics to restore the function of downregulated tumor suppressor miRNAs, and antagomirs or locked nucleic acid (LNA)-based inhibitors to silence overexpressed oncogenic miRNAs. For instance, the miR-122 inhibitor miravirsen has been evaluated in clinical trials for hepatitis C, demonstrating the feasibility of systemic miRNA targeting. Delivery remains a significant challenge for miRNA-based therapies, with ongoing research focusing on nanoparticle carriers, exosomes, and tissue-specific delivery systems [78]. Furthermore, the pleiotropic nature of miRNAs necessitates careful design to minimize off-target effects.

7.4 Cosmetic and medical interventions

The intersection of medical research and esthetic practice has facilitated the advancement of therapeutic interventions that address both health and appearance [79]. Cosmetic procedures are increasingly acknowledged not only for their esthetic value but also for their potential therapeutic benefits in dermatology, reconstructive medicine, and mental well-being [80, 81]. Medical-grade interventions such as botulinum toxin injections, dermal fillers, laser therapies, and microneedling are employed to treat conditions such as facial palsy, acne scarring, rosacea, and hyperhidrosis [82]. Platelet-rich plasma (PRP) therapy, initially developed for wound healing, has found applications in alopecia, skin rejuvenation, and musculoskeletal conditions [79]. Concurrently, emerging technologies like regenerative esthetics (e.g., stem cell-based therapies, growth factor serums) and minimally invasive body contouring are increasingly blurring the distinction between cosmetic care and medical treatment. Personalized approaches that consider genetic and epigenetic profiles are also being explored to optimize outcomes and minimize adverse effects. As consumer demand and clinical efficacy continue to converge, the integration of cosmetic and medical approaches is poised to expand, underscoring the importance of regulatory frameworks and evidence-based practice [80].

8. Clinical implications and future directions

8.1 Early detection and preventive strategies

Investigating the epigenetic modifications associated with solar lentigines (SL) facilitates advancements in proactive dermatological care [83]. Epigenetic biomarkers, including DNA methylation signatures, histone modification patterns, and microRNA profiles, have the potential to detect subclinical photoaging early, before the appearance of visible symptoms. A study by Peng, Liu [26] states that the early identification of individuals predisposed to SL may be achieved through noninvasive sampling methods, such as skin swabs or tape stripping, in conjunction with high-throughput epigenomic assays. Preventive strategies could be more effectively tailored by integrating epigenetic risk profiles with data on environmental exposure [84]. For instance, individuals exhibiting UV-sensitive methylation patterns in genes related to pigmentation or oxidative stress could receive guidance on enhanced photoprotection, lifestyle adjustments, and early topical interventions. Sunscreen formulations enriched with epigenome-stabilizing agents, such as polyphenols or retinoids, may become integral components of daily care regimens customized to epigenetic risk [26].

8.2 Personalized dermatology and epigenomic profiling

As precision medicine becomes increasingly integrated into dermatology, epigenomic profiling presents substantial potential for customizing therapeutic and cosmetic interventions for solar lentigines (SL) and broader photoaging disorders [85]. The incorporation of individual epigenetic data into dermatological practice may facilitate the differentiation of overlapping pigmentary conditions, such as melasma and SL, guide treatment intensity, and predict responses to various modalities, including chemical peels, laser therapy, and topical agents [86]. Furthermore, the co-profiling of transcriptomic and epigenomic data could reveal novel therapeutic targets, such as silenced antioxidant genes or upregulated pro-pigmentation pathways. Inhibitors or activators of specific histone-modifying enzymes, such as histone deacetylases (HDACs) and histone acetyltransferases (HATs), as well as DNA methyltransferases, may provide targeted approaches to reverse pigmentation and rejuvenate the extracellular matrix [86]. The future may witness the emergence of "epigenetic skincare," involving customized serums or topical formulations designed to modulate specific skin gene expression patterns altered by UV exposure [87].

9. The somatologist's role in a current treatment method

A Somatologist, also referred to as a Dermal Therapist or Advanced Aesthetician, is a highly skilled skin care expert who serves as a link between medical dermatology and esthetic treatments [88]. Although they are not medical doctors, their expertise in advanced, noninvasive techniques and skin health science makes them helpful in addressing complex issues such as solar lentigines [88]. Their responsibilities go beyond merely applying treatments, encompassing thorough analysis, client education, and the development of long-term strategic plans.

9.1 Introductory approach: Analysis, triage, and education

The work of a Somatologist starts with a comprehensive skin evaluation, often employing sophisticated imaging devices such as VISIA or a Wood's Lamp to evaluate the extent of photodamage [89]. An essential initial step in this procedure is triage, which involves identifying any suspicious lesions and promptly referring them to a dermatologist to exclude the possibility of malignancies like melanoma. Following this, the somatologist's primary responsibility is to educate clients. They explain how prolonged exposure to UV rays epigenetically changes pigment-producing cells, resulting in ongoing hyperpigmentation. This educational groundwork is essential for establishing realistic expectations, emphasizing that while treatments can eliminate current spots, they cannot remove this inherent cellular memory. This is supported by practical guidance on inclusive sun protection (encompassing UVA, UVB, and visible light) and the adoption of a pre-treatment conditioning routine. By employing tyrosinase inhibitors and retinoids, this preparatory stage enhances the skin's receptiveness to advanced therapies, boosting effectiveness and reducing risks such as post-inflammatory hyperpigmentation [90].

9.2 Cutting-edge therapeutic interventions

A somatologist might carry out or assist with advanced treatments selected for their effectiveness in addressing the unique biological aspects of photodamage [90, 91]. These treatments encompass:

- *Picosecond Lasers:* This technology delivers ultrashort energy pulses, creating a photoacoustic effect that shatters pigment with minimal heat. This makes it a safe and effective option for all skin types, significantly reducing the risk of thermal damage.

- *BroadBand Light (BBL):* BBL not only removes melanin in lentigines but also has been shown to modulate gene expression in aging skin, making it more closely resemble that of younger skin. This directly addresses the epigenetic component of photoaging, providing both corrective and rejuvenative benefits.

- *Fractional Non-Ablative Lasers:* By creating microscopic treatment zones, these lasers stimulate collagen production and expel old, pigmented cells, improving both skin tone and texture.

- *Microneedling with Targeted Actives:* This technique creates microchannels in the skin, dramatically enhancing the delivery of potent ingredients like tranexamic acid. This allows the active to penetrate deeply and inhibit key pathways in melanin production.

9.3 Long-term management and prevention of recurrence

One of the most vital roles of a somatologist is crafting an advanced, long-term maintenance strategy. Since solar lentigines are influenced by epigenetic factors and tend to reappear, a single treatment session is not enough [57]. The somatologist formulates a complementary homecare routine using state-of-the-art cosmeceuticals with components like cysteamine or thiamidol, which block several stages of the pigment production process. This continuous, proactive method is crucial for inhibiting pigment formation, preventing recurrence, and ensuring that the results achieved in the clinic are maintained over time.

10. Interdisciplinary approaches in skin aging management

Addressing solar lentigines and photoaging necessitates a multidisciplinary approach that integrates dermatology, somatology, molecular biology, cosmetic science, bioinformatics, and behavioral health [38, 92]. Collaborative efforts among clinicians, researchers, and data scientists are essential for deciphering complex epigenetic interactions and developing user-friendly, clinically validated platforms for real-time skin monitoring [92, 93]. Furthermore, integrative health approaches, such as nutritional epigenomics and psycho-dermatology, may offer supplementary strategies for managing chronic photoaging. Dietary components with established epigenetic activity (e.g., curcumin, sulforaphane, and omega-3 fatty acids) could play supportive roles in modulating systemic oxidative stress and skin inflammation [80, 81]. Mental health interventions that mitigate chronic stress may help prevent cortisol-induced epigenetic dysregulation of skin repair mechanisms. Collectively, these advanced strategies pave the way for a more nuanced, biologically informed model of skin aging and pigmentary disorder management, where prevention, personalization, and interdisciplinarity converge to enhance outcomes for patients affected by solar lentigines.

11. Conclusion

Solar lentigines (SL) are a clear manifestation of photoaging and represent far more than superficial hyperpigmentation. This review highlights that their formation is deeply rooted in significant molecular disruptions caused by epigenetic mechanisms. Prolonged exposure to ultraviolet (UV) radiation and the consequent oxidative stress lead to enduring changes in DNA methylation, histone modifications, and noncoding RNAs. These changes foster a dysfunctional cellular environment that encourages ongoing melanogenesis, chronic low-grade inflammation, and accelerated cellular aging, partly through a senescence-associated secretory phenotype (SASP). This molecular "memory" accounts for the persistence and recurrence of SL, making it a crucial model for understanding the profound nature of skin aging. This advanced insight is paving the way for a new wave of targeted therapies. Epigenetic modulators, such as sirtuin activators and regulatory microRNAs, hold great potential by addressing the underlying dysregulation rather than just the visible symptoms. By acting at the molecular level, these innovative treatments could restore cellular balance, reverse epigenetic marks, and diminish the factors driving pigmentation and inflammation. This shift towards personalized, biologically informed treatments represents a significant advancement in both medical and cosmetic dermatology, promising more effective and lasting results. Ultimately, managing a condition with such a complex, epigenetically driven basis necessitates an equally sophisticated and interdisciplinary clinical approach. While dermatologists play a vital role in providing medical diagnoses and performing advanced treatments to clear existing lesions, this only addresses part of the issue. The somatologist is a crucial partner in implementing a long-term strategic plan. Their expertise in patient education, behavioral change, and holistic care is essential for managing environmental triggers and lifestyle factors that sustain the condition. By developing comprehensive care plans that include rigorous sun protection, antioxidant support, and lifestyle adjustments, the somatologist ensures that the results achieved in the clinic are maintained. This collaborative partnership effectively addresses the persistent nature of solar lentigines, leading to healthier skin and more successful and enduring outcomes for the client.

Author details

Nomakhosi Mpofana[1*], Mokgadi Ursula Makgobole[1] and Pavitra Pillay[2]

1 Department of Somatology, Durban University of Technology - Ritson Campus, Durban, KwaZulu-Natal, South Africa

2 Department of Biomedical and Clinical Technology, Faculty of Health Sciences, Durban University of Technology, Durban, South Africa

*Address all correspondence to: nomakhosim@dut.ac.za

References

[1] Tang X et al. Current insights and future perspectives of ultraviolet radiation (UV) exposure: Friends and foes to the skin and beyond the skin. Environment International. 2024:108535

[2] Verma A et al. Skin protection from solar ultraviolet radiation using natural compounds: A review. Environmental Chemistry Letters. 2024;**22**(1):273-295

[3] Dorosz A et al. The impact of environmental factors on skin and tissue ageing: Mechanisms, effects, and preventive strategies. Journal of Education, Health and Sport. 2025;**79**:58282-58282

[4] Savita S. The impact of climate change on dermatological conditions: Analyzing the effects of UV exposure and pollution. Scholar's Digest: Journal of Dermatology. 2025;**1**(1):59-78

[5] Abati S et al. Differential diagnosis of pigmented lesions in the oral mucosa: A clinical based overview and narrative review. Cancers. 2024;**16**(13):2487

[6] Hara Y, Shibata T. Characteristics of dermal vascularity in melasma and solar lentigo. Photodermatology, Photoimmunology & Photomedicine. 2024;**40**(2):e12953

[7] Mulawa ME, Niczyporuk M. Skin pigmentation changes, causes and methods of their elimination. Polish Journal of Applied Sciences. 2024;**9**(2):28-34

[8] Zhang M et al. Exploring mechanisms of skin aging: Insights for clinical treatment. Frontiers in Immunology. 2024;**15**:1421858

[9] Tusiimire J, Josephine M, Nantege M. The Human Skin, its Ageing Process, and Current Anti-Ageing Cosmeceutical Products. Abakaliki, Nigeria: Academic Journals; 2025

[10] Serna Higuita LM. Population Based and Clinical Epidemiologic Studies on Different Forms of Skin Cancer. Tübingen, Germany: Universität Tübingen; 2024

[11] Tumsutti P, Rojhirunsakool S. Effects of Topical Corticosteroids, Topical Corticosteroids under Occlusion, and Topical Brimonidine on the Prevention of Postinflammatory Hyperpigmentation after Q-Switched 532-Nm Nd: YAG Laser Treatment of Solar Lentigines. Bangkok, Thailand: Srinakharinwirot University; 2024

[12] Niska K et al. Cytotoxicity of ZnO nanoparticles in human melanocyte cells in the presence or absence of UV radiation: A preliminary comparative study with TiO2 nanoparticles. Toxicology In Vitro. 2025;**106**:106051

[13] Papaccio F et al. Persistent β-hexachlorocyclohexane exposure impacts cellular metabolism with a specific signature in Normal human melanocytes. Cells. 2024;**13**(5):374

[14] Barnes BM et al. Epigenetics and ultraviolet radiation: Implications for skin ageing and carcinogenesis. Skin Health and Disease. 2024;**4**(6):e410

[15] Kaya VO, Adebali O. UV-induced reorganization of 3D genome mediates DNA damage response. Nature Communications. 2025;**16**(1):1376

[16] Scalera C. Investigations of the UV-Induced DNA Damage Response in Human Cells and Zebrafish Embryos. Mainz, Germany: Johannes Gutenberg-Universität Mainz; 2024

[17] Sedley L. The Epigenetics and Biological Clock of Skin Cancer. Basel, Switzerland: MDPI; 2025

[18] Abubakar M. Overview of skin cancer and risk factors. International Journal of General Practice Nursing. 2024;**2**(3):42-56

[19] Konstantinou E, Longange E, Kaya G. Mechanisms of senescence and anti-senescence strategies in the skin. Biology. 2024;**13**(9):647

[20] Del Bino S, Duval C, Bernerd F. Clinical and biological characterization of skin pigmentation diversity and its consequences on UV impact. International Journal of Molecular Sciences. 2018;**19**(9):2668

[21] Hanel A, Carlberg C. Skin colour and vitamin D: An update. Experimental Dermatology. 2020;**29**(9):864-875

[22] Choi W et al. Molecular and histological characterization of age spots. Experimental Dermatology. 2017;**26**(3):242-248

[23] Hasegawa K et al. Increased blood flow and vasculature in solar lentigo. The Journal of Dermatology. 2016;**43**(10):1209-1213

[24] Sivaraman Siveen K et al. Vascular endothelial growth factor (VEGF) signaling in tumour vascularization: Potential and challenges. Current Vascular Pharmacology. 2017;**15**(4):339-351

[25] Jeong J et al. Multi-system-level analysis reveals differential expression of stress response-associated genes in inflammatory solar lentigo. International Journal of Molecular Sciences. 2024;**25**(7):3973

[26] Peng Q et al. Genetic variants in telomerase reverse transcriptase contribute to solar lentigines. Journal of Investigative Dermatology. 2023;**143**(6):1062-1072 e25

[27] Pollefliet C et al. Morphological characterization of solar lentigines by in vivo reflectance confocal microscopy: A longitudinal approach. International Journal of Cosmetic Science. 2013;**35**(2):149-155

[28] Salminen A, Kaarniranta K, Kauppinen A. Photoaging: UV radiation-induced inflammation and immunosuppression accelerate the aging process in the skin. Inflammation Research. 2022;**71**(7):817-831

[29] Ma J et al. Autophagy plays an essential role in ultraviolet radiation-driven skin photoaging. Frontiers in Pharmacology. 2022;**13**:864331

[30] Wang M et al. Autophagy: Multiple mechanisms to protect skin from ultraviolet radiation-driven photoaging. Oxidative Medicine and Cellular Longevity. 2019;**2019**(1):8135985

[31] Zhong X et al. Role of autophagy in skin photoaging: A narrative review. Medicine. 2024;**103**(8):e37178

[32] Nakamura M et al. Environment-induced lentigines: Formation of solar lentigines beyond ultraviolet radiation. Experimental Dermatology. 2015;**24**(6):407-411

[33] Vogeley C et al. Role of the aryl hydrocarbon receptor in environmentally induced skin aging and skin carcinogenesis. International Journal of Molecular Sciences. 2019;**20**(23):6005

[34] Kerns ML et al. Pathogenic and therapeutic role for NRF2 signaling in ultraviolet light–induced skin pigmentation. JCI Insight. 2020;**5**(20):e139342

[35] Roman ÁC et al. The aryl hydrocarbon receptor in the crossroad of signalling networks with therapeutic value. Pharmacology & Therapeutics. 2018;**185**:50-63

[36] Wardyn JD, Ponsford AH, Sanderson CM. Dissecting molecular cross-talk between Nrf2 and NF-κB response pathways. Biochemical Society Transactions. 2015;**43**(4):621-626

[37] He F, Ru X, Wen T. NRF2, a transcription factor for stress response and beyond. International Journal of Molecular Sciences. 2020;**21**(13):4777

[38] OpenAI. Diagrammatic Illustration of the Various Factors Involved in the Process of Skin Aging. 2025. ChatGPT (Version GPT-5). Available from: https://chatgpt.com/c/6899df79-82d8-8328-a2f0-04e46ad09a02 [Accessed: August 11, 2025]

[39] Henshall DC, Kobow K. Epigenetics and epilepsy. Cold Spring Harbor Perspectives in Medicine. 2015;**5**(12):a022731

[40] Avery-Kiejda KA. Switching off Cancer: Is there a Role for Epigenetics? Basel, Switzerland: MDPI; 2021. p. 1272

[41] Horvath S et al. Epigenetic clock for skin and blood cells applied to Hutchinson Gilford progeria syndrome and ex vivo studies. Aging (Albany NY). 2018;**10**(7):1758

[42] Wagner W. The link between epigenetic clocks for aging and senescence. Frontiers in Genetics. 2019;**10**:303

[43] Weidner CI, Wagner W. The epigenetic tracks of aging. Biological Chemistry. 2014;**395**(11):1307-1314

[44] Wan DC, Wang KC. Long noncoding RNA: Significance and potential in skin biology. Cold Spring Harbor Perspectives in Medicine. 2014;**4**(5):a015404

[45] Rorteau J et al. Functional integrity of aging skin, from cutaneous biology to anti-aging strategies. Medecine Sciences: M/S. 2020;**36**(12):1155-1162

[46] Hussein RS et al. Influences on skin and intrinsic aging: Biological, environmental, and therapeutic insights. Journal of Cosmetic Dermatology. 2025;**24**(2):e16688

[47] Liu Z et al. Telomeres in skin aging. Biogerontology. 2025;**26**(2):83

[48] Haykal D et al. Unlocking longevity in aesthetic dermatology: Epigenetics, aging, and personalized care. International Journal of Dermatology. 2025

[49] Hüls A et al. Lentigine formation in Caucasian women—Interaction between particulate matter and solar UVR. Journal of Investigative Dermatology. 2019;**139**(4):974-976

[50] Yang Y et al. UVB drives different stages of epigenome alterations during progression of skin cancer. Cancer Letters. 2019;**449**:20-30

[51] Takeshima H, Ushijima T. Accumulation of genetic and epigenetic alterations in normal cells and cancer risk. npj Precision Oncology. 2019;**3**(1):7

[52] Zhou L, Lim HW, Mi Q-S. Epigenetics. In: Vitiligo. Cham, Switzerland, Springer Nature; 2019. pp. 253-264

[53] Xu Q et al. Transcriptomic analysis of coding genes and non-coding RNAs reveals complex regulatory networks underlying the black back and white belly coat phenotype in chinese Wuzhishan pigs. Genes. 2019;**10**(3):201

[54] Jiang L et al. Ganoderma lucidum polysaccharide reduces melanogenesis by inhibiting the paracrine effects of keratinocytes and fibroblasts via IL-6/STAT3/FGF2 pathway. Journal of Cellular Physiology. 2019;**234**(12):22799-22808

[55] Qiu W, Chuong CM, Lei M. Regulation of melanocyte stem cells in the pigmentation of skin and its appendages: Biological patterning and therapeutic potentials. Experimental Dermatology. 2019;**28**(4):395-405

[56] Hossain MR et al. Diversified stimuli-induced inflammatory pathways cause skin pigmentation. International Journal of Molecular Sciences. 2021;**22**(8):3970

[57] Kim M et al. Senescent fibroblasts in melasma pathophysiology. Experimental Dermatology. 2019;**28**(6):719-722

[58] Jakhar R, Crasta K. Exosomes as emerging pro-tumorigenic mediators of the senescence-associated secretory phenotype. International Journal of Molecular Sciences. 2019;**20**(10):2547

[59] Dańczak-Pazdrowska A et al. Cellular senescence in skin-related research: Targeted signaling pathways and naturally occurring therapeutic agents. Aging Cell. 2023;**22**(6):e13845

[60] Victorelli S et al. Senescent human melanocytes drive skin ageing via paracrine telomere dysfunction. The EMBO Journal. 2019;**38**(23):e101982

[61] Gao P et al. Lysine Carboxymethyl Cysteinate, as a topical glutathione precursor, protects against oxidative stress and UVB radiation-induced skin damage. Antioxidants. 2025;**14**(5):606

[62] Duval C et al. A chronic pro-inflammatory environment contributes to the physiopathology of actinic lentigines. Scientific Reports. 2024;**14**(1):5256

[63] Ali SA, Naaz I. Current challenges in understanding the story of skin pigmentation—Bridging the morpho-anatomical and functional aspects of mammalian melanocytes. Muscle Cell and Tissue. 2015;**1**:262-285

[64] Upadhyay PR, Ho T, Abdel-Malek ZA. Participation of keratinocyte- and fibroblast-derived factors in melanocyte homeostasis, the response to UV, and pigmentary disorders. Pigment Cell & Melanoma Research. 2021;**34**(4):762-776

[65] Chandrasekaran A. Redox-Dependent Calcium-Mediated Signaling Networks That Control the Senescence-Associated Secretory Phenotype. Amsterdam, Netherlands, Elsevier; 2017

[66] Fu C et al. Roles of inflammation factors in melanogenesis. Molecular Medicine Reports. 2020;**21**(3):1421-1430

[67] Natarajan VT et al. IFN-γ signaling maintains skin pigmentation homeostasis through regulation of melanosome maturation. Proceedings of the National Academy of Sciences. 2014;**111**(6):2301-2306

[68] Velarde MC, Demaria M. Targeting senescent cells: Possible implications for delaying skin aging: A mini-review. Gerontology. 2016;**62**(5):513-518

[69] Chin T et al. The role of cellular senescence in skin aging and age-related skin pathologies. Frontiers in Physiology. 2023;**14**:1297637

[70] Zhang L, Lu Q, Chang C. Epigenetics in health and disease. Epigenetics in Allergy and Autoimmunity. 2020;**1253**:3-55

[71] Mu S et al. Autoimmune disease: A view of epigenetics and therapeutic targeting. Frontiers in Immunology. 2024;**15**:1482728

[72] Bosch-Presegue L, Vaquero A. Sirtuins in stress response: Guardians of the genome. Oncogene. 2014;**33**(29):3764-3775

[73] Carafa V et al. Sirtuin functions and modulation: From chemistry to the clinic. Clinical Epigenetics. 2016;**8**:1-21

[74] Ding Y-N et al. Roles of Sirtuins in cardiovascular diseases: Mechanisms and therapeutics. Circulation Research. 2025;**136**(5):524-550

[75] Fiorentino F et al. Sirtuin modulators: Past, present, and future perspectives. Future Medicinal Chemistry. 2022;**14**(12):915-939

[76] Tyagi N et al. Exploiting nanotechnology for the development of microRNA-based cancer therapeutics. Journal of Biomedical Nanotechnology. 2016;**12**(1):28-42

[77] Dasgupta I, Chatterjee A. Recent advances in miRNA delivery systems. Methods and Protocols. 2021;**4**(1):10

[78] Wang H et al. Recent progress in microRNA delivery for cancer therapy by non-viral synthetic vectors. Advanced Drug Delivery Reviews. 2015;**81**:142-160

[79] White C et al. Platelet-rich plasma: A comprehensive review of emerging applications in medical and aesthetic dermatology. The Journal of Clinical and Aesthetic Dermatology. 2021;**14**(11):44

[80] Fedorchenko Y. Platelet-rich plasma in anti-aging and aesthetic medicine. Anti-Aging Eastern Europe. 2024;**3**(4):168-174

[81] Trovato F et al. Advancements in regenerative medicine for aesthetic dermatology: A comprehensive review and future trends. Cosmetics. 2024;**11**(2):49

[82] Arora G, Arora S. Medical aesthetics–current trends and a review of its applications. Indian Dermatology Online Journal. 2023;**14**(3):309-319

[83] Yamada T et al. UV irradiation-induced DNA hypomethylation around WNT1 gene: Implications for solar lentigines. Experimental Dermatology. 2019;**28**(6):723-729

[84] Yang X et al. Integrated bioinformatics analysis reveals diagnostic biomarkers and immune cell infiltration characteristics of solar Lentigines. Clinical, Cosmetic and Investigational Dermatology. 2024;**17**:79-88

[85] Julie ZY, Friedland MH, McGee JS. Epigenetics and precision medicine in skin diseases. In: Epigenetics in Precision Medicine. Amsterdam, Netherlands: Elsevier; 2022. pp. 193-221

[86] Ghosh K, O'Neil K, Capell BC. Histone modifiers: Dynamic regulators of the cutaneous transcriptome. Journal of Dermatological Science. 2018;**89**(3):226-232

[87] Haykal D. Leveraging single nucleotide polymorphism profiling for precision skin care: How SNPs shape individual responses in cosmetic dermatology. Journal of Cosmetic Dermatology. 2025;**24**(1):e16750

[88] Mpofana N, Maitland Griffiths CE, Cordelia Dlova N. The feasibility of an interdisciplinary approach on the management of psoriasis in South Africa. Alternative Therapies in Health and Medicine. 2022;**28**(2):58-64

[89] Nicholas Brownstone N. Comparing Devices to Assess Facial Pigmentary and Inflammatory Conditions. United States, MJH Life Sciences; 2024

[90] Nkwanyana S. An Investigation of the Professional Relationship between Somatologists and Medical Professionals Practicing Non-invasive Aesthetic and Anti-Ageing Medicine in eThekwini. Durban, South Africa, Durban University of Technology (DUT); 2015

[91] Jaiswal S, Jawade S. Microneedling in dermatology: A comprehensive review of applications, techniques, and outcomes. Cureus. 2024;**16**(9):e70033

[92] Rinnerthaler M, Bischof J, Streubel, MK, Trost A, Richter K. Oxidative stress in aging human skin. Biomolecules. 2015;**5**(2):545-589

[93] Goorochurn R et al. Biological processes in solar lentigo: Insights brought by experimental models. Experimental Dermatology. 2016;**25**(3):174-177

Chapter 4

Systemic Blood Changes in Skin Hyperpigmentation – Correction Possibilities

Maria Glushkova

Abstract

Acquired hyperpigmentation is widespread in the population and significantly affects the quality of life of patients. It is known that one of the clinical signs of skin hyperpigmentation is localized hyperkeratosis in the lesion, associated with a high level of cell proliferation and cell saturation with melanin. Cellular proliferation and hyperkeratosis are associated with increased local metabolism rates. The phenomenon of skin hyperpigmentation is accompanied by a restructuring of blood cell metabolism aimed at preserving oxygen and energy homeostasis in skin structures. The obtained data indicate a redistribution of oxygen in cellular structures and tissues, which is accompanied by a significant increase in lactate concentration and the formation of local tissue hypoxia.

Keywords: hyperpigmentation, tissue hypoxia, lipoproteins, melasma, post-inflammatory hyperpigmentation, melanin

1. Introduction

Acquired skin hyperpigmentation is widespread in the population and significantly affects the quality of life. Many factors play an important role in the development of these conditions. One of the most important is inflammation in response to ultraviolet (UV) radiation, disruption of the body's antioxidant system, photoaging, hypersensitivity of melanocytes (MCs), excessive production of melanin, genetic predisposition, taking photosensitizing drugs, hormonal dysfunction, previous skin damage, and a number of other poorly understood mechanisms [1].

Melasma is the result of increased activity of MCs, which are influenced by a number of factors. These include hereditary hypersensitivity of MCs, photodamage, hormonal status changes, metabolic disorders, liver and gastrointestinal tract diseases, and the use of photosensitizers. With regard to post-inflammatory hyperpigmentation, the duration and intensity of previous inflammation and skin damage are crucial [2].

Melanogenesis is one of the complex phenotypes of an organism's adaptation to the environment. Melanin is the cell's defense against genotoxic damage. This natural

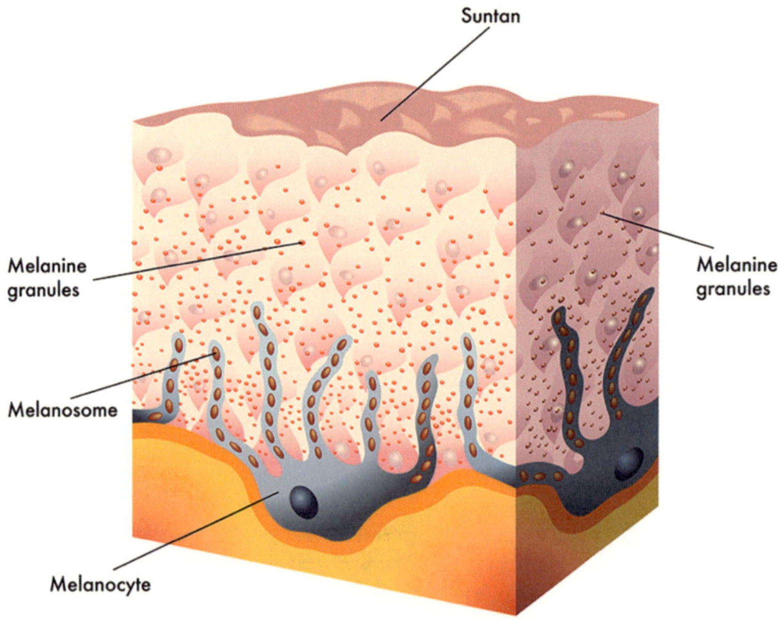

Figure 1.
The schematic representation of melanin and melanocytes in the skin.

heteropolymer acts as a broadband UV absorber, antioxidant, and radical scavenger. UVA is a factor in natural selection. Disruption of melanogenesis is thought to be a major risk factor for melanoma and other cancers [3].

Melanin is an amino acid derivative produced by MCs through a series of enzymatic reactions using tyrosinase as a substrate. Human skin and hair color are also closely related to melanin, so understanding the mechanisms and proteins that produce melanin is very important. There are many proteins involved in the process of melanin expression (**Figure 1**).

In the typical human epidermis, 40 keratinocytes (KCs) cluster around 1 MC, and the MC unites with the KC. KCs' connective dendritic branches act as conduits for mature melanosome trafficking to the KC (Moreiras et al., 2021).

MCs produce melanosomes, which are then transported to adjacent KCs, ascending in layers and eventually becoming visible in the human epidermis **Figure 2**. In this process, many ions interact with proteins to affect the process, some of which influence the production of melanosomes and some of which regulate their transport [4].

And some protein families not only affect the generation of melanin small bodies but also play a role in the transport of melanin bodies.

In addition to changing human skin color and hair color, melanin also has some very valuable advantages. Melanin not only absorbs UV and visible light but also has free radical scavenging and antioxidant capacity; it protects cells from toxic damage and mitigates the damaging effects of UV on cellular macromolecules. This prevents DNA damage and pathogenic mutations caused by UV radiation on the skin [5].

Melanin, derived from tyrosine and other similar phenolic chemicals, forms the widely dispersed phenolic biopolymer. According to the different synthetic

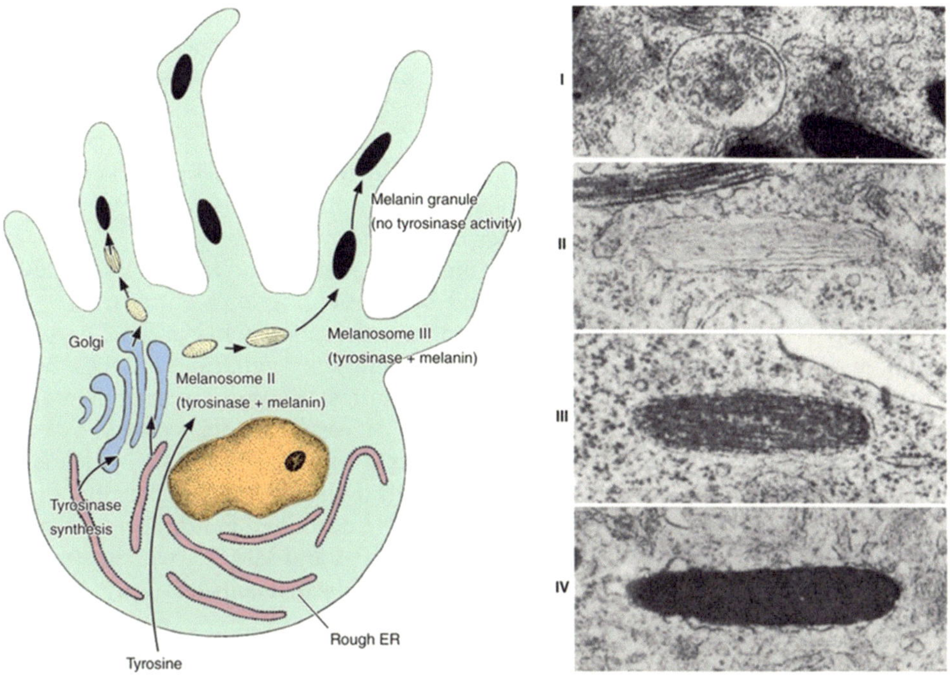

Figure 2.
The scheme of the melanocyte. The schematic representation of the melanocyte. The structure of the melanicyte.

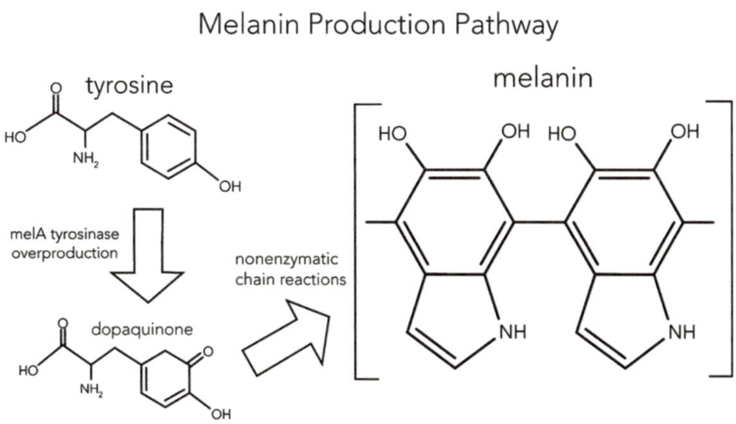

Figure 3.
The synthesis of melanin. The biochemical basics. The melanin production pathway.

pathways and intermediate metabolites, melanin can be mainly divided into eumelanin, pheomelanin, and allomelanin, and its sources can include bacteria, fungi, plants, or animals (Wakamatsu and Ito, 2023) (**Figure 3**).

L-tyrosine is converted by tyrosinase to L-3,4-dihydroxyphenylalanine (L-DOPA), and L-DOPA to dopaquinone. Dopaquinone then proceeds through a sequence of reduction and oxidation processes to yield 5,6-dihydroxyindole and 5,6-dihydroxyindole-2-carboxylic acid, which are the building blocks of eumelanin.

Pigmentation is considered to be the result of interactions between MCs and neighboring cells, such as KCs and fibroblasts, which change significantly with aging. UV irradiation activates fibroblasts to release melanogenic growth factors, including hepatocyte growth factor (HGF), KC growth factor (KGF), stem cell factor (SCF), and endothelin-1 (ET-1), which act together on MCs both directly and indirectly through KCs, promoting hyperpigmentation [6].

Due to the development of molecular biology, genetics, and immunology, new data on the pathogenesis of the disease have been emerging in recent years. According to modern concepts, persistent inflammation is the key and primary mechanism by which the production of pro-inflammatory cytokines induces the process of melanogenesis. At the moment, the manifestations of hyperpigmentation are equated with such a concept as photo-aging. An essential role is played by the mechanism of activation of the transcription factor AP-1 in fibroblasts, which is a central inducer of impaired collagen homeostasis in the skin and is a key link in the pathogenesis of both photo- and chrono-aging. The described factor also activates the expression of genes encoding the enzymes MMP-1 and MMP-3, which stimulate the degradation (fragmentation) of matrix fibrils of dermal collagen [7].

2. Study

Acquired skin hyperpigmentations are pathogenetically associated with increased MC activity. However, the issue of the formation of molecular mechanisms of occurrence is not fully disclosed. AHH are widespread in the population and significantly affect the quality of life of patients. It is known that one of the clinical signs of skin hyperpigmentation is localized hyperkeratosis in the lesion focus, associated with a high level of cell proliferation and cell saturation with melanin. A large amount of energy and substrates is required to maintain increased cellular metabolism. Therefore, we decided to demonstrate these interactions using the example of our research.

2.1 Objective

To study systemic changes in blood counts in skin hyperpigmentation compared to the control group and their changes after treatment.

2.2 Methods

The patient database was formed using MS Excel spreadsheets, version 19.0 (manufactured by Microsoft, USA). Statistical analysis was performed using the IBM SPSS Statistical software, version 26.0 (manufactured in the USA). All the writing of the work, the creation of the database, and the statistical analysis of the data were carried out on a personal computer.

Quantitative indicators were evaluated for compliance with the normal distribution law using the Shapiro–Wilk criterion (for samples with fewer than 50 women) and the Kolmogorov–Smirnov criterion (for samples with more than 50 women). At a significance level of $p > 0.05$, it was assumed that the samples obeyed the normal distribution law; in the opposite case, it was assumed that the samples did not obey this law.

Quantitative indicators with a normal distribution were described using arithmetic averages (M) and standard deviations (SD) in the form of M ± SD. In the absence of a normal distribution, quantitative data were described using the median (Me) and the lower and upper quartiles (25% and 75% [Q1; Q3]). The minimum and maximum values of each sample were also described.

The comparison of quantitative indicators in the groups, in pairs, for independent samples was carried out using the parametric t-Student criterion (for samples that obey the NPR) and the nonparametric Mann–Whitney criterion (for samples that do not obey the NPR). For dependent samples (before and after treatment), the Student's t-test was applied for dependent samples, and in cases where the samples did not obey the NPR, the Wilcoxon criterion was applied.

In the case of multiple comparative analysis of quantitative indicators (three or more groups), the nonparametric Kruskal–Wallis criterion was used (for samples that do not obey the normal distribution law), followed by a posteriori pairwise comparative analysis adjusted for likelihood (mainly using the Bonferroni correction). If the samples obeyed the normal distribution law, then the analysis of variance (ANOVA) method was used for multiple analysis.

To describe parametric (categorical) data, absolute values (number of people) and relative values (frequency of occurrence, %) were used.

A comparative analysis of categorical data was carried out using Fisher's exact criterion and/or Pearson's chi-square (χ^2).

When comparing dependent samples (before/after) for categorical data, a comparative analysis was performed using the McNemar criterion.

In all cases where $p < 0.05$ was present, the differences were considered statistically significant; otherwise, the differences were not statistically significant.

The aim of the study was to identify systemic changes in blood parameters in patients with PHC Acquired skin hyperpigmentations before and after treatment, as well as to assess their possible contribution to the mechanisms of formation of skin hyperpigmentation.

The study was open-ended, randomized, prospective, comparative, and controlled. It was conducted between 2023 and 2024 and included 85 women.

All patients were divided into two groups: the control group (25 people, 29.4%), which consisted of healthy women, and the main group (60 people, 70.6%), which consisted of sick women. The main group was divided into two subgroups: melasma (31 women, 51.7%) and post-inflammatory hyperpigmentation (29 women, 48.3%).

At the first stage, a multifactorial cluster analysis was performed on patients with hyperpigmentation to identify the form of the disease and collect anamnestic data, as well as laboratory tests conducted before treatment for selected indicators [**Table 1**].

All patients were examined, including their hormonal status. They were somatically healthy and did not take any medications.

At the second stage, patients with melasma underwent topical and hardware treatment aimed at the fragmentation of melanin granules and the inhibition of melanogenesis. The topical treatment included the daily use, for 12 weeks, of cosmetic lightening creams (day and night) containing a combination of active ingredients: glabridine, anthrafolide, and lysine azelate, and represented a non-ablative effect of Nd:Yag 1,064 nm in the nanosecond range with Q-Switch modulation. The same topical therapy was used for patients with PVH, but the hardware treatment was

Indicators	Groups		Statistical significance level, p^* *correct*
	Main	Control	
Age, years	41.88 ± 1.45	41.84 ± 1.57	0.926
Height, cm	16.676 ± 3.61	16.652 ± 4.93	0.845
Weight, kg	65.80 ± 6.28	63.08 ± 5.96	0.123
Body mass index, kg/m^2	23.70 ± 2.56	22.81 ± 2.52	0.221

Notes: The table was compiled by the authors.
** Statistical significance according to Student's criterion for independent samples.*

Table 1.
Mean values (M ± SD) of certain indicators for individuals in the compared groups, if comparable.

different. Non-ablative exposure of Nd:Yag with 1,064 nm laser radiation in the microsecond range was performed. The duration of treatment did not differ between the subgroups and was 12 weeks. The intervals between exposures were two weeks in both subgroups, for a total of six.

The material for the study was blood serum and red blood cells.

Lactate, PVC, and 2,3-DPH were detected in erythrocytes.

Lipoproteins of various classes, collagen, MMP-1, MMP-3, R–IL-6, IL-6, NOS-3, HOI-1, SH, cartilaginous glycoprotein-39, γ(IP-10) – inducible interferon protein, were determined in blood serum.

Blood, as a multifunctional tissue that integrates all body environments, reflects the changes occurring in all tissues and organs, and red blood cells, representing a universal membrane model, accurately reflect the changes occurring in other cellular structures.

The erythrocyte, closely contacting and interacting with all tissues, reflects the changes occurring in the body – both physiological and pathological – through its structure and metabolic restructuring.

Taking into account the role of the circulatory system in oxygenation homeostasis, we evaluated the metabolic regulation of the oxygen transport function of erythrocytes based on the determination of such parameters as lactate, PBC, and 2,3-DPG.

Blood, as a polyfunctional tissue integrating all the organism's environments, reflects changes occurring in all tissues and organs, and erythrocytes, representing a universal membrane model, quite often reflect changes in other cellular structures.

Since oxygen utilization by the skin tissue is an important metabolic link providing homeostasis, we studied the peculiarities of the gas transport function of erythrocytes in the blood of patients with hyperpigmentation and in the control group.

The process of hyperpigmentation formation is pathogenetically related to the disturbance of microcirculation, which leads to changes in oxygen transport [2, 3].

In this aspect, the functional state of erythrocytes in skin hyperpigmentation and in the control group was studied.

3. Results

It was of interest to study changes in this function by measuring the concentration of lactic acid, pyruvic acid (PVA), and the level of 2,3-diphosphoglycerate (2,3-DPG) (**Figures 4**, **5**).

DOI: http://dx.doi.org/10.5772/intechopen.1013671

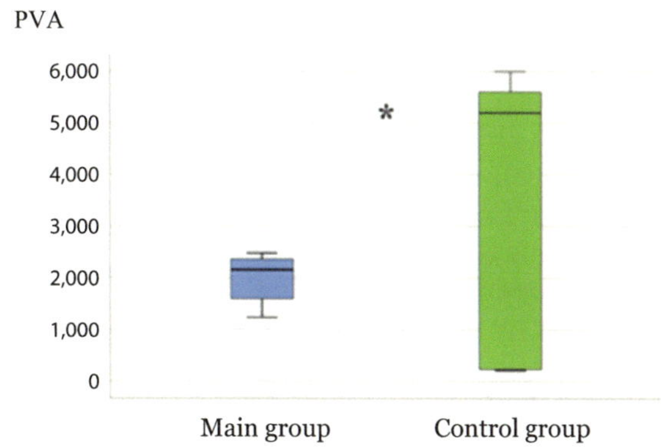

Figure 4.
Comparison of the levels of pyruvic acid in the erythrocytes of venous blood in the main and control groups.

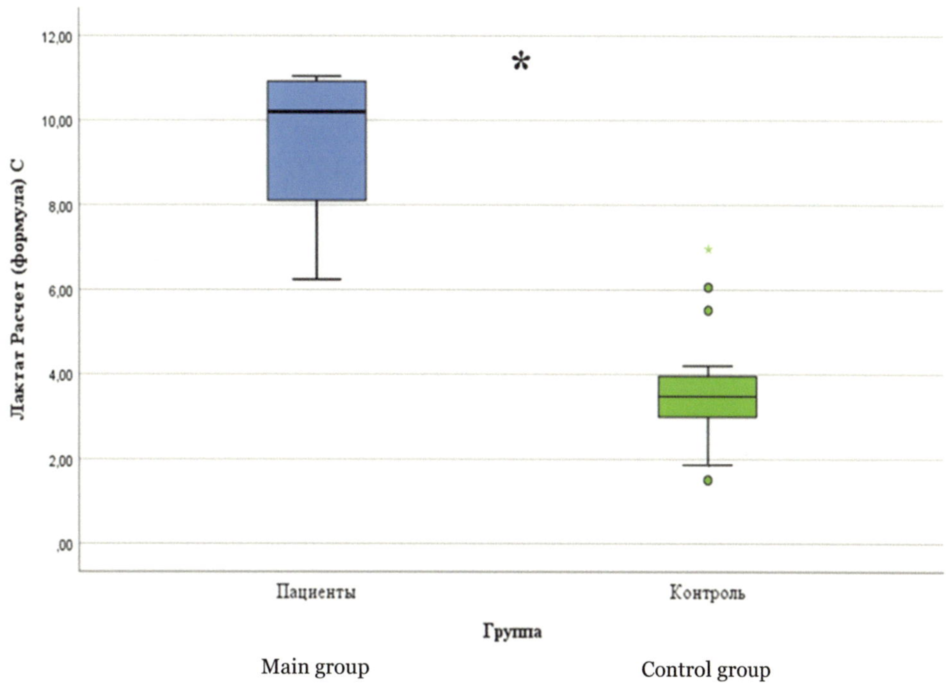

Figure 5.
Comparison of lactate levels in red blood cells of venous blood in the main and control groups.

It was found that, in the red blood cells of women in the clinical group with skin hyperpigmentation, the concentration of PVA was significantly reduced by 86% (the differences were statistically significant, $p = 0.03$ according to the Mann–Whitney criterion) compared with the control group. At the same time, there was an increase in lactate levels by 167.4% (the differences were statistically significant, $p = 0.02$ according to the Mann–Whitney criterion) relative to the control group.

A decrease in the level of PVA in the erythrocytes of patients with hyperpigmentation reflects the activation of the rate of anaerobic glycolysis, which may affect the gas transport function of erythrocytes.

However, it should be noted that the level of 2,3-DPG in the main group did not significantly differ from the control but tended to increase.

These unidirectional changes from anaerobic glycolysis were characteristic of both study groups (melasma and PIH). Obviously, the increased concentration of lactate, against the background of maintaining a constant level of 2,3-DPH, indicates that part of the oxygen is used not for tissue respiration but for enhanced synthesis of melanin and saturation of neighboring KCs with it. In other words, there is a change in the priority of oxygen consumption toward the synthesis of melanin (**Figures 6**, 7).

Lactate levels decreased by 68.82%. The concentration of 2,3-DPG decreased by 43.24%.

Under the current metabolic situation, increased melanin synthesis requires the participation of a large amount of oxygen.

However, it seemed interesting to us to study different classes of lipoproteins and their possible contribution to the process of melanogenesis.

Thus, the level of cholesterol in patients with hyperpigmentation was statistically significantly different from the control by 18.64% **Figure 8**.

A higher TG (triacylglycerides) content was found – by 18.1% in the main group.

The number of VLDL (very low-density lipoproteins) decreased by 18.13%, and LDL (low-density lipoproteins) decreased by 44.93%.

Summarizing the results obtained, it can be noted that the phenomenon of skin hyperpigmentation is accompanied by a restructuring of blood cell metabolism aimed at maintaining oxygen and energy homeostasis in skin structures. To ensure the formation of hyperpigmentation and melanogenesis as a process, it is necessary to supply a sufficient amount of plastic and energy substrates. This leads to an

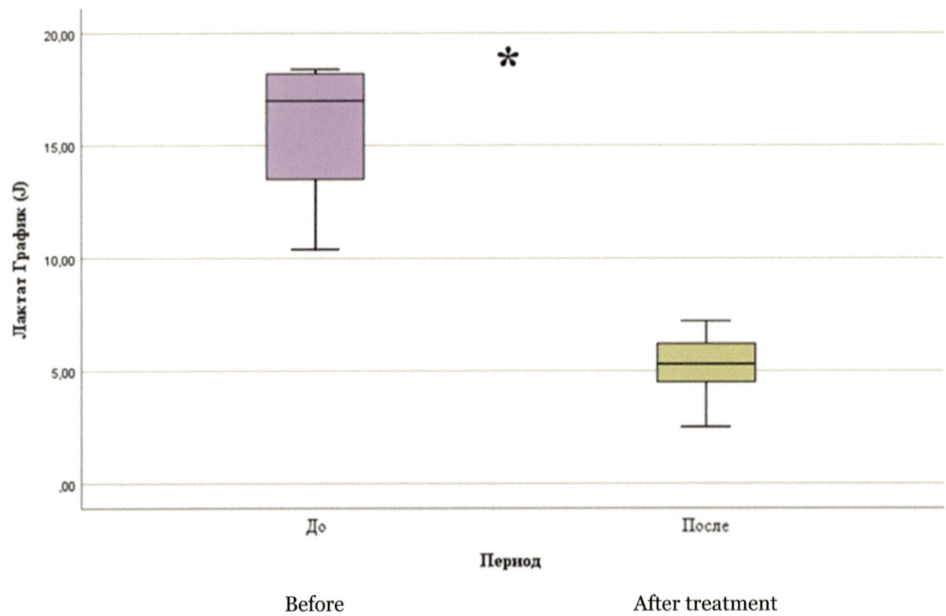

Figure 6.
Comparison of lactate levels in red blood cells of venous blood in the main group before and after treatment (Nd: YAG laser 1,064 nm).

DOI: http://dx.doi.org/10.5772/intechopen.1013671

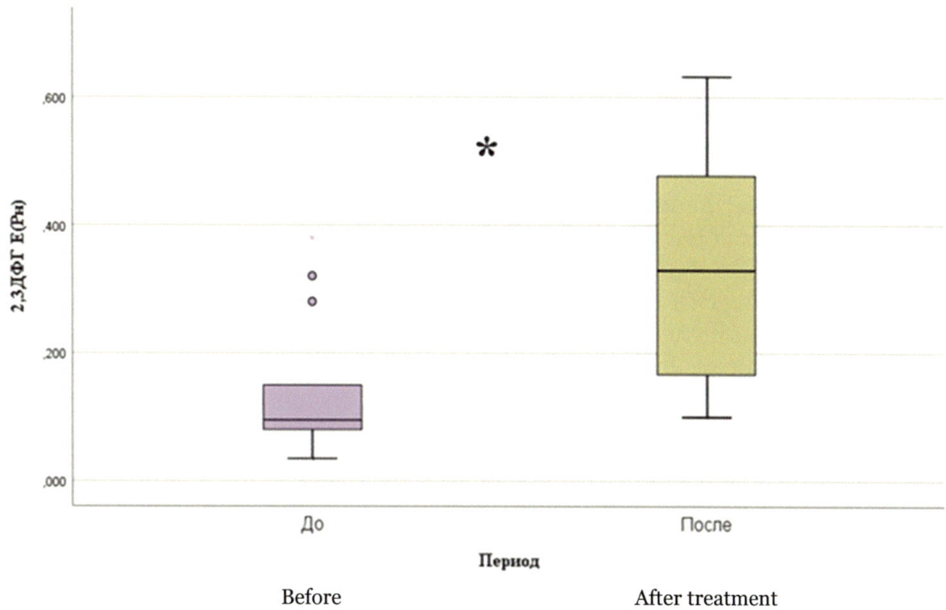

Figure 7.
The changing the name will distort the meaning of our research and the re Comparison of 2,3-DPG concentration in red blood cells of venous blood in the main group before and after treatment (Nd:YAG laser 1,064 nm).

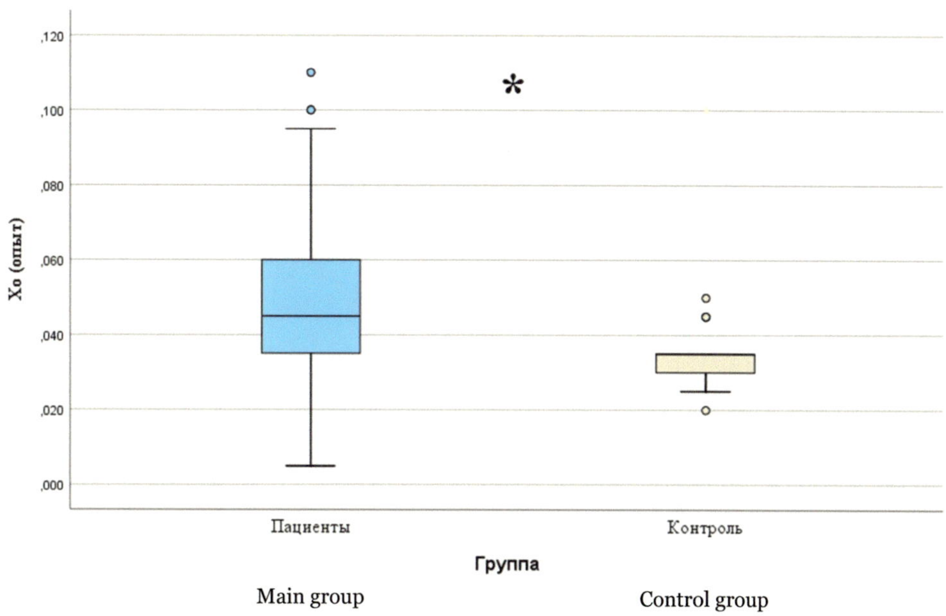

Figure 8.
Comparison of cholesterol levels in the serum of venous blood in the main and control groups.

uneven redistribution of oxygen and fatty acids supplied to the skin, as well as a change in the metabolism of the intercellular matrix of the skin.

The physiological role of lipoproteins in ensuring the transport of cholesterol and triglycerides to peripheral tissues is important in conditions of intensive proliferation and metabolic activity of epidermal cells. Hyperactivity of MCs and KCs in hyperpigmentation foci requires increased intake of both energy substrates and components for building cell membranes and melanin synthesis. In this regard, the elevated levels of low-density lipoproteins (LDL) and very low-density lipoproteins (VLDL) recorded in the group before treatment can be considered a compensatory reaction to increased lipid and structural metabolism in the skin. After treatment, positive dynamics were observed – a decrease in OH, TG, and LDL levels with a simultaneous increase in HDL, which indicates normalization of the level of lipid transport forms and confirms the systemic effect of the therapy **Figure 9**.

At the same time, the TG level decreased by 9.57% after treatment.

At the same time, after treatment, the cholesterol level decreased by 23.21% **Figure 10**.

The LDL level decreased by 82.77% after treatment. HDL levels increased by 18.6% after treatment **Figure 11**.

Since the process of hyperpigmentation is associated with a change in the structure of connective tissue, the dermal basis of which is collagen and elastin, it seemed interesting to study such indicators as collagen, MMP-1, and MMP-3.

The level of collagen was higher in the main group by 72.41% [**Figure 12**].

The level of MMP-1 was statistically significantly different in the patients of the control group and was 156.25% higher. [**Figure 13**]. Reduction of collagenase witnesses active collagen synthesis. The MMP-3 level was 42.86% higher before treatment.

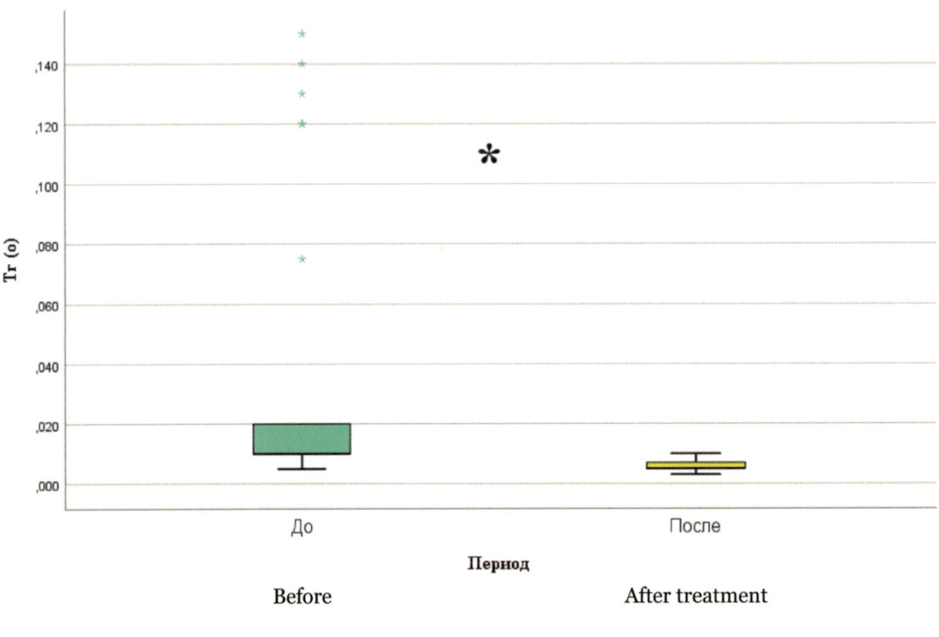

Figure 9.
Comparison of triacylglyceride levels in the serum of venous blood in the main group before and after treatment.

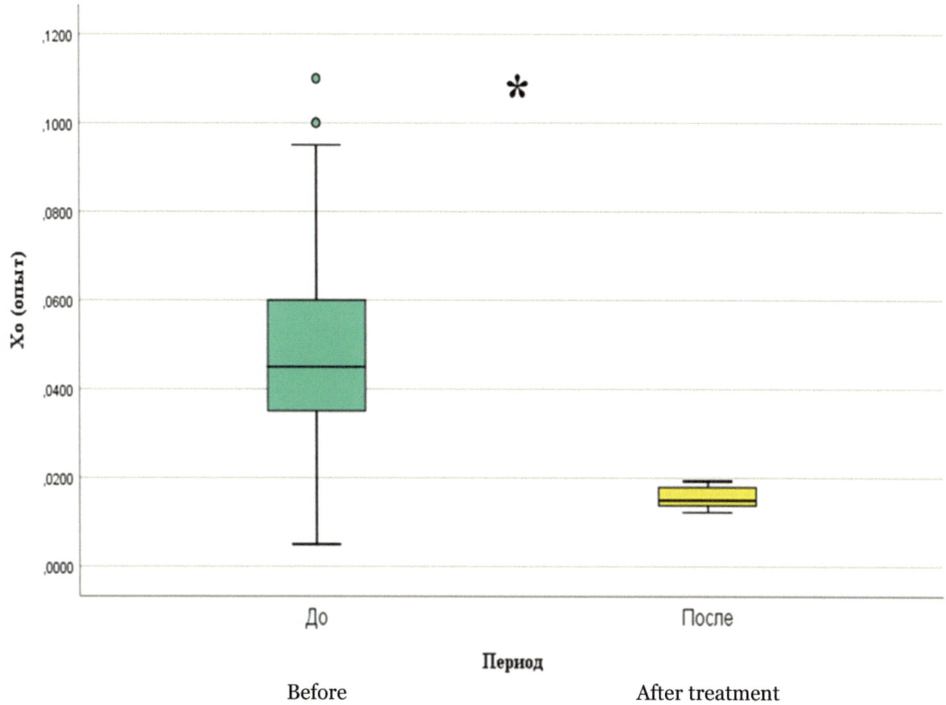

Figure 10.
Comparison of cholesterol levels in the serum of venous blood in the main group before and after treatment.

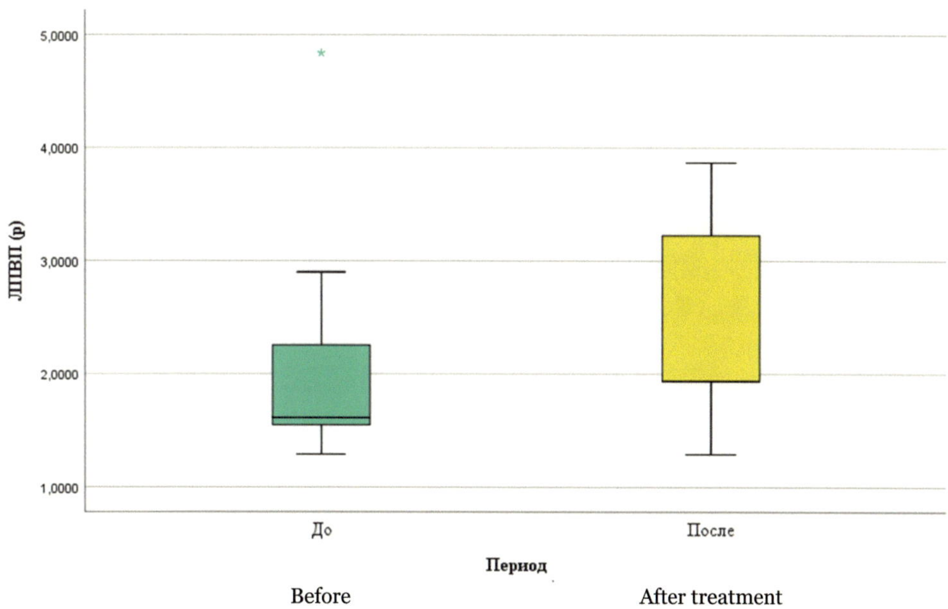

Figure 11.
Comparison of high-density lipoprotein (HDL) levels in the serum of venous blood in the main group before and after treatment.

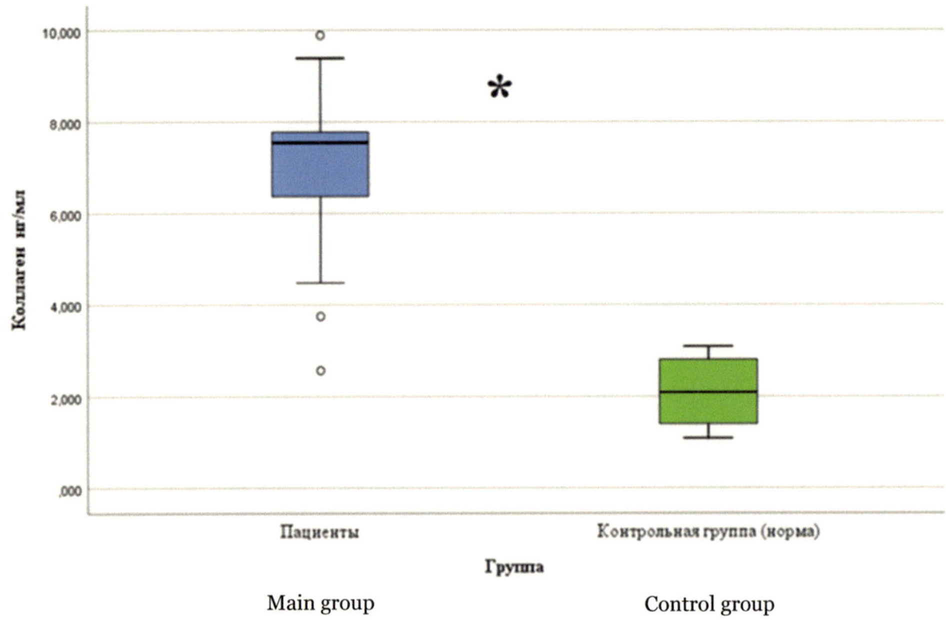

Figure 12.
The level of collagen in the blood serum of patients in the main and control groups.

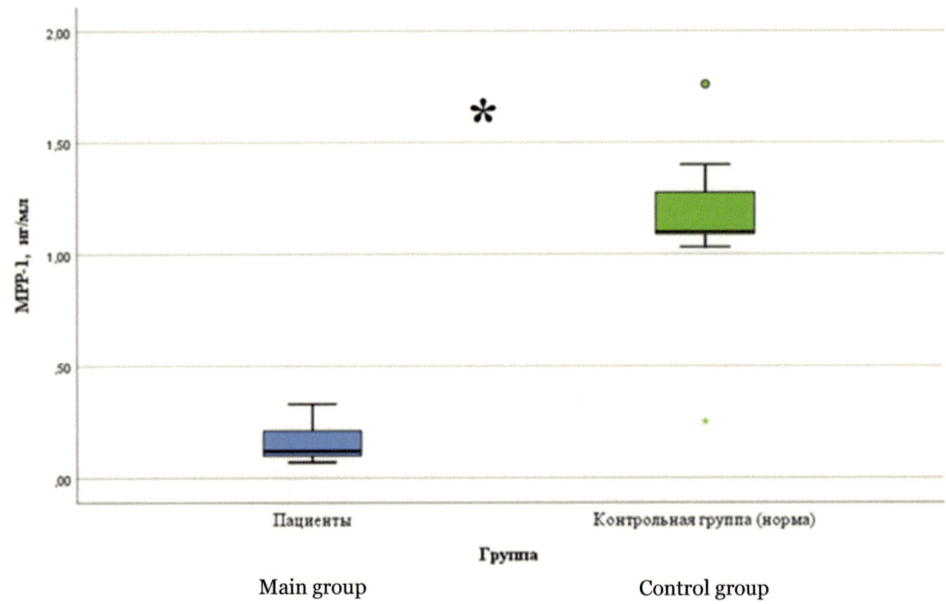

Figure 13.
The level of metalloprotease-1 (MPP-1) in the blood serum of patients in the main and control groups.

At the same time, the TG level decreased by 9.57% after treatment. The LDL level decreased by 82.77% after treatment. HDL levels increased by 18.6% after treatment.

Lactate levels decreased by 68.82%. The concentration of 2,3-DPG increased by 43.24%.

During the study, it was found that γ(IP-10)-inducible interferon protein (quantitative) showed statistically significant differences before and after treatment in the main group. After treatment, it decreased by 85.86%.

4. Discussion

The activation of melanin synthesis, associated with hyperpigmentation and increased sloughing of KCs, is accompanied by even greater oxygen consumption, resulting in its uneven redistribution between cell structures and metabolic pathways.

The results obtained indicate a change in the local oxygenation of pathological tissue with the involvement of metabolic life support systems, which include a circulating erythrocyte pool that triggers both damage mechanisms and the formation of protective and adaptive reactions, implemented at the molecular membrane level and aimed at ensuring tissue homeostasis and adaptation of the cell population as a whole.

The decrease in PVA concentration toward the increase of lactate in erythrocytes of patients with hyperpigmentation indicates the presence of tissue hypoxia, which leads to impaired microcirculation in the pathological focus. In the main clinical group, there was a significant increase in the concentration of lactate, which may indicate the presence of tissue hypoxia in the pathogenesis of hyperpigmentation.

In patients, after treatment, the lactate concentration approached the reference values. The increase in lactate concentration can be considered an adaptive reaction to the process of hypoxia in the area of hyperpigmentation.

Since the process of hyperpigmentation is accompanied by cell proliferation, synthesis, and saturation with melanin of the MCs themselves and all surrounding KCs, a large amount of plastic material is required, aimed at building cell membranes.

A decrease in the concentration of pyruvate, toward with an increase in lactate in the erythrocytes of patients with hyperpigmentation, indicates an uneven distribution of oxygen in the skin and a violation of microcirculation in the pathological focus. Namely, it suggests a change in the priority of oxygen consumption, not only for tissue respiration but also to ensure enhanced melanogenesis. In the main clinical group, there was a significant increase in lactate concentration, which may indicate the conversion of pyruvate to lactate. In patients of the main clinical group, after treatment, the lactate concentration approached the reference values. An increase in lactate concentration can be considered an adaptive reaction to the process of increased oxygen consumption by tissues and cells during hyperpigmentation.

Violation of the gas transmission and energy function of erythrocytes in patients with hyperpigmentation of the main group before treatment indicates activation of anaerobic glycolysis under conditions of tissue hypoxia. These changes are caused by impaired microcirculation in the dermis, especially in the hyperpigmentation zone, where oxygen consumption is increased as a result of melanogenesis. Hypoxia, in this case, may be associated with either focal vascular spasm, overload of the capillary bed, or an unequal redistribution of oxygen between metabolically active cells.

After the course of treatment, the lactate concentration approached the norm and equaled the values in the control group, while the level of pyruvate did not significantly change, and the level of 2,3-DPG decreased. The changes that have occurred may indicate the restoration of microcirculation and normalization of tissue respiration. The stabilization of indicators after therapy demonstrates not only the local but also the possible systemic effect of therapy on the restoration of metabolic homeostasis.

Metabolism in red blood cells is essentially limited to anaerobic glycolysis and the hexose monophosphate shunt, with glucose serving as the main source of energy. In the process of glycolysis, a glucose molecule is broken down into two lactic acid molecules. The energy output is two molecules of ATP. The ATP formed during glycolysis is primarily a substrate for Na^+/K^+-ATPase, which supports the membrane potential of red blood cells. Additionally, ATP supports the glycolysis process itself, as the hexokinase and phosphofructokinase reactions are energy-dependent. The final reaction of anaerobic glycolysis is the reduction of pyruvate to lactate, catalyzed by lactate dehydrogenase. Lactic acid is metabolized mainly in the kidneys, heart, and liver, and is only rarely excreted in the urine. Lactate represents a kind of dead end in metabolism, as the only possible way to utilize it is to convert lactic acid back into pyruvate. This process is achievable by reversing the lactate dehydrogenase reaction under aerobic conditions. Most of the pyruvate is oxidized to CO_2 and acetyl-CoA. The oxidation of acetyl-CoA in the tricarboxylic acid cycle results in the formation of 36 (or 38) ATP molecules. In the presence of oxygen deficiency, carbohydrate metabolism in the cell is severely disrupted, leading to the accumulation of lactic acid and a sharp decrease in the energy capacity of the cell [4].

Exposure to ultraviolet sunlight initiates inflammatory reactions in the skin, which lead to increased activity of MCs and the formation of hyperpigmented areas. With systemic inflammation, there is an increase in the lipid content and a change in the profile of lipoproteins in the blood, which has a typically stereotypical protective character. This increase is due to the fact that lipoproteins reduce the toxicity of lipopolysaccharides and act as free radical scavengers, inhibiting peroxidation processes. That is, adaptive reactions at the level of lipid metabolism play an important role in protecting the skin from damage caused by inflammation and solar radiation.

Obviously, a high level of LDL is associated with the active intake of cholesterol esters into the epidermal layer, which are hydrolyzed to their monomers, used to build cell membranes, and higher fatty acids (HFA) are actively used to ensure the energy consumption of the pathological process.

According to recent studies, the process of photosterization and pigmentation is associated with metabolic reprogramming provided by the oxidation of fatty acids. Switching in metabolic processes may be associated with a marked increase in dermal white adipose tissue (dWAT) in aging skin. Cutaneous adipocytes undergo cyclic processes of dedifferentiation and redirection, which lead to an increased release of free fatty acids into the extracellular space during differentiation [Khabarov V. N. Collagen, Elastin, Hyaluronic Acid in Molecular Cosmetology]. One of the critically important factors influencing these processes is the protein adiponectin, which regulates multiple activities through endocrine, paracrine, or autocrine mechanisms [Cayo A., Segovia R., Venturini W. et al. mTOR Activity and Autophagy in Senescent Cells, a Complex Partnership]. Oxidative modifications of phospholipids in aging dermal fibroblasts have also been identified, which are associated with the secretory phenotype characteristic of aging. Probably, the interrelation of these processes is reflected in our research.

It is known that lipid peroxidation products (POL) play a key role in the pathogenesis of various dermatological disorders, including acquired skin hyperpigmentation. Peroxidation of the lipid bilayer leads to damage to cell membranes, which, in turn, causes their destruction and the release of lysosomal enzymes. These enzymes activate the formation of vasoactive substances such as histamine and bradykinin. As a result, an inflammatory reaction occurs, which contributes to an even greater depletion of the energy potential of cells, especially under conditions of insufficient oxygenation. These mechanisms can accelerate tissue damage and worsen the symptoms of hyperpigmentation. Inflammation causes a proatherogenic lipid metabolism disorder, and lipid metabolism disorders can cause the development of pro-inflammatory disorders [8].

An increase in this indicator underlies chronic inflammation and high cellular activity. It is known to be secreted by chondrocytes, synovial cells, neutrophils, and activated macrophages. It correlates with the degree of inflammation. What correlates with the criteria indexes?

The constant rearrangement of the main macromolecular components leads to the necessary changes in the cellular environment. The processes of rearrangement of the intercellular substance are an important component of physiological tissue remodeling.

5. Conclusion

The formation of skin pigmentation is considered a physiological mechanism in response to inflammation, mainly associated with ultraviolet radiation. The general strategy of the inflammatory process under normal regulation and dysregulation shows differences. It seems necessary to further study systemic adaptation mechanisms in dysregulation in patients with skin hyperpigmentation, as well as to reveal predictors contributing to its formation. The feasibility of studying the systemic biochemical profile in patients with skin hyperpigmentation will allow the development of optimal drug correction schemes.

The conducted research served as the basis for optimizing the algorithm of instrumental diagnostics, a differential approach to therapy characterized by high cost-effectiveness and shorter treatment times.

Given the chronic nature of the course of melasma and the risk of exacerbation, we consider it necessary to provide supportive treatment in an intermittent regimen, with an interval of three months in the first year of follow-up.

The developed combined treatment regimen for patients with melasma and post-inflammatory hyperpigmentation of the skin helps reduce pigmentation in the lesion, is an effective and safe method, and offers a differential approach and versatility in application.

Author details

Maria Glushkova
Scientific Director of the Department of Medical Cosmetology at the DAVINCI Clinic, Rostov-on-Don, Russia

*Address all correspondence to: mariaglushkova06@gmail.com

References

[1] Kubanova AA, Manturova NE, Gallyamova YA. Manual on cosmetology. ANO Publishing House "Scientific Review". 2020;728

[2] Potekaev NN, Avram MR, Tsao S, Tannous Z, Avram MM. Atlas of Cosmetic Dermatology/translated from English. Publishing House Binnom; 2013. p. 295

[3] Burylina OM, Karpova AV. Cosmetology: Clinical Guide. Moscow: Geotar-Media; 2018. p. 744

[4] Torres-Alvarez B, Mesa-Garza IG, Castanedo-Cazares JP, Fuentes-Ahumada C, Oros-Ovalle C, Navarrete-Solis J, Moncada B. Histochemical and immunohistochemical study in melasma: Evidence of damage in the basal membrane. The American Journal of Dermatopathology. 2011;**33**:291–295

[5] Kim NH, Lee CH, Lee AY. H19 RNA downregulation stimulated melanogenesis in melasma. Pigment Cell & Melanoma Research. 2010;**23**:84–92

[6] Cardinali G, Kovacs D, Giglio MD, Cota C, Aspite N, Amantea A, Girolomoni G, Picardo M. A kindred with familial progressive hyperpigmentation-like disorder: Implication of fibroblast-derived growth factors in pigmentation. European Journal of Dermatology. 2009;**19**:469–473

[7] Kim EH, Kim YC, Lee ES, Kang HY. The vascular characteristics of melasma. Journal of Dermatological Science. 2007;**46**:111–116

[8] Klimov AN, Parfenova NS, Golikov YP. To the 100th anniversary of the creation of the cholesterol model of atherosclerosis. Biomedical Chemistry. 2012;**58**(1):5–11

Chapter 5

Perspective Chapter: Pigmentation Disorders of Aging Retina – Prevention and NonInvasive Management Options

Sanda Jurja, Ticuta Negreanu-Pirjol, Mihaela Cezarina Mehedinti, Ana Maria Dascalu, Florentina Nicoleta Roncea, Maria-Andrada Hincu and Bogdan-Stefan Negreanu-Pirjol

Abstract

Pigment disorders of both aging skin and retina involve many common mechanisms. A better understanding of such mechanisms might lead to effective prevention and noninvasive therapy strategies applicable to both locations of pigmentary disorders. The direct consequence of such pigmentary disorders involving the retinal tissue generates age-related macular degeneration (AMD), the leading cause of vision loss in the elderly, which occurs as a progressive loss of macular pigments. Oxidative stress on retinal pigment is nowadays exacerbated by environmental factors such as chronic ultraviolet (UV) exposure, pollution, toxic heavy metal accumulation, and amplified by climate change. Increased risks of damaging effects urge proactive preventive strategies and therapies. Nutritional antioxidant supplementation has emerged as a key preventive approach. Clinical studies in AMD patients indicate that long-term Xanthophyll carotenoid supplementation can slow the progression of degeneration and vision loss. Beyond these, a variety of plant-derived supplements have demonstrated significant *in vitro/in vivo* antioxidative activity, with protective anti-aging effects. This comprehensive paradigm, linking antioxidative nutrition, environmental risk mitigation, and medical therapies, exemplifies a modern translational strategy to reduce oxidative damage and improve outcomes in retinal aging pigment disorders.

Keywords: pigmentation disorders, nutritional supplements, aging, retina, antioxidant activity, maculopathy

1. Introduction

In the next decades, the prevalence of retinal degenerative diseases, especially those that involve the retinal pigment epithelium (RPE), is expected to rise drastically [1, 2]. In this article, we have conducted a comprehensive investigation into the mechanisms that drive pigment metabolism dysregulation within the aging retina, with a focus on noninvasive procedures and prevention strategies.

However, the most visible manifestation of human aging is skin aging, frequently perceived as a marker of the senescence process. Both the macroscopic aspect and cellular/molecular structure are changing. There are two different types of skin aging that occur, each with characteristic features: chronological aging and photoaging. Of these two types, the latter is more commonly represented by pigmentary abnormalities, mostly similar to the retinal pigment abnormalities in terms of formation and metabolic mechanisms. Moreover, the issue of lysosomal lipofuscin deposits and glycogen granules in aging skin cells has been noticed, similar to those found in the aging retina [3–5]. A diversity of agents, such as sun exposure, genetics, and microcirculation, as well as some histopathological aspects regarding vascular proliferation, have been identified as being correlated with pigmentary disorders in both the skin and retina.

Aging entails stress in both the skin and retina. The free radical mechanism reveals that oxidative metabolism, with excessive and continuous production of reactive oxygen species (ROS), determines tissue damage.

Another surprising similarity between skin and retina regarding pigmentary aging disorders consists of the abundance of biomolecules such as lipids, proteins, and DNA. These molecules are targeted by oxidative aggression, followed by intracellular damage [6–8].

Considering the above and returning to retinal pigment disorders, we examine the degradation of melanin, the accumulation of lipofuscin, and alterations in pigment granule composition as hallmark features of RPE aging. Epigenetic dysregulation, including DNA methylation, micro-RNA (miRNA) imbalance, and histone modification, proves to be a pivotal mechanism underlying these pigmentary shifts [9, 10]. The study proposes a novel clinical framework based on the link between molecular profiling and advanced retinal imaging procedures, such as fundus autofluorescence (FAF) and optical coherence tomography (OCT), in order to detect early subclinical pigmentary changes before anatomical damage appears.

We explore and document noninvasive therapeutic approaches: epigenetic modulators such as resveratrol, curcumin, and folate, alongside miRNA-based therapies and light-mediated interventions [10–14]. A stratified prevention algorithm is proposed, integrating epigenetic assays with multimodal imaging to better classify patients into risk tiers and guide personalized interventions. Moreover, the role of the ocular surface microbiome is taken into consideration, offering new diagnostic and therapeutic opportunities. Ultimately, this chapter reframes pigment imbalance as a modifiable and detectable early event in retinal degeneration. By combining insights from molecular biology, nutritional science, microbiome research, and imaging diagnostics, we lay the groundwork for a shift from reactive to proactive care.

2. Noninvasive strategies and epigenomic insights in retinal aging

As populations age, disorders related to the RPE are considered significant contributors to visual decline [1, 2]. This structure, a single pigmented cell layer, plays a vital role in metabolic support, photo protection, and removal of photoreceptor outer segments. Its structural integrity is essential for maintaining visual acuity and preserving normal retinal function [15, 16]. Another key factor that must be considered is the role of oxygen in this process. A growing body of evidence highlights the damaging impact of reactive oxygen intermediates (ROIs) on ocular tissue aging and degenerative pathologies, leading to the broader acceptance of the concept of oxidative stress [12, 13, 17].

During aging, RPE-associated cells accumulate pigment granules such as lipofuscin, melanosomes, and complex melanolipofuscin granules [16, 18]. These molecules result from lysosomal digestion of photoreceptor debris and may occupy up to 30% of the RPE cytoplasmic volume. Recent studies show that light exposure, particularly within the blue-green spectrum, promotes the generation of ROS, which degrade melanin within adjacent melanolipofuscin granules [18, 19]. This degradation is associated with the progressive loss of melanin, impairing antioxidant defense mechanisms and increasing oxidative stress within the RPE [16, 18].

Furthermore, it has been suggested that this complex mechanism may underlie negative visual outcomes in a significant percentage of elderly patients suffering from vision impairment [1, 9].

Beyond pigment granule dynamics, epigenetic mechanisms are increasingly recognized as regulators of RPE cell fate and pigment metabolism [9–11]. DNA methylation, miRNA expression, and histone acetylation are considered pivotal in gene regulation, cell differentiation, and adaptive responses to environmental stressors [9, 10, 20]. Despite growing recognition of the RPE's role in visual decline associated with elderly patients [1, 2], the specific molecular regulation of granule dynamics is not yet completely understood. While melanin degradation and lipofuscin accumulation have been extensively studied in the aging RPE [15, 16, 18], the regulatory networks, particularly at the epigenetic and transcriptional levels, remain largely unexplored. A compelling example includes the role of specific genes, miRNAs, or chromatin states in governing the synthesis, transport, and degradation of melanin structures and how these mechanisms are altered with age.

Additionally, there is a notable lack of noninvasive options and preventive strategies aimed specifically at reversing or delaying pigment imbalance in the aging retina. Current clinical management continues to focus primarily on late-stage disease rather than preserving RPE function during the predegenerative phase [1, 2]. Moreover, the potential for modulating epigenetic regulators noninvasively, such as through diet, light exposure, or naturally occurring chromatin-modifying compounds, remains under-investigated.

2.1 Integrating imaging, epigenetics, and nutritional therapies for retinal pigment preservation

To address these gaps, a holistic approach is required. The first challenge involves molecular profiling of the aging RPE, especially at the epigenomic level, which may uncover key regulators of pigment metabolism and granule turnover [9, 10, 20]. Secondly, *in vivo* technologies, such as FAF, should be further developed to allow longitudinal and noninvasive tracking of pigmentary changes [21, 22]. This article reviews the current knowledge of age-related pigmentary pathology in the retina, explores the involvement of epigenetic mechanisms in RPE degeneration, and highlights potential noninvasive interventions to prevent or mitigate pigmentary disorders. By bridging practical prevention strategies, such as light-filtering technologies, epigenetic-targeted therapies, and detailed molecular understanding, we aim to provide a comprehensive foundation for future research and clinical innovation focused on maintaining retinal pigmentation during aging.

Age-related changes, such as melanin degradation and lipofuscin accumulation, are well-documented [15, 16, 19, 21]; however, the associated regulatory networks, particularly those involving epigenetic and transcriptional control, are not yet fully understood in aging human tissue.

A model proposed by Grigoryan and Markitantova highlights that epigenetic plasticity within RPE cells plays a crucial role in determining their fate during regeneration phases [9]. In vertebrate species capable of retinal regeneration, the RPE maintains an open chromatin landscape, permitting transdifferentiation into retinal neurons. In contrast, mammalian RPE is characterized by repressive chromatin modifications, which constrain its regenerative potential. The authors suggest that these same epigenetic barriers may also influence pigment metabolism, although this dimension remains insufficiently explored [9].

In parallel, emerging findings on emdoplasmic reticulum (ER)–melanosome contact sites offer promising insights into intracellular pigment transport and turnover, a process increasingly implicated in aging but still lacking validation as a clinical target [23]. A study on tyrosinase expression in optic nerve degeneration has also shown that transcriptional stress responses can influence pigment biosynthesis, hinting at broader regulatory interactions beyond the retina itself [24]. These knowledge gaps limit both the ability to detect early subclinical changes and the development of targeted interventions. Should pigment imbalance be confirmed as an initiating factor in retinal degeneration rather than a downstream effect, early detection and correction strategies would become essential.

To address these issues, this chapter outlines several clinical priorities. First, epigenomic profiling of aging human RPE is necessary to identify master regulators of pigment metabolism. Second, advanced imaging techniques, such as FAF and OCT, should be used to detect pigment imbalance before structural atrophy becomes evident. Third, noninvasive therapeutic options, including dietary epigenetic modulators, miRNA-based interventions, and light-mediated therapies – must be developed to preserve melanin integrity and limit oxidative pigment degradation.

Although studies like those of Grigoryan and Markitantova have demonstrated distinct chromatin accessibility patterns in regenerative versus degenerative RPE states, they have yet to focus on pigment-regulation-specific genes such as TYR, OCA2, or LAMP2 [9]. Other recent work reinforces the view that age is a major factor influencing the epigenome–metabolism interface in these cells [25, 26]. Signaling pathways such as VEGF and BMP have been characterized between the RPE and choroid in senescence, but no comprehensive epigenetic mapping of pigment-related genes has been completed to date. Even the classic histological markers of aging RPE are insufficiently connected to upstream genomic or epigenomic regulators, leaving essential mechanistic links unexplored.

Further research has started to explore how ER–melanosome contact sites, recently identified in mammalian RPE, might regulate pigment trafficking via transcriptional control. Human iPSC-derived RPE organoid models have demonstrated that pigment biosynthesis pathways can be reactivated by inhibiting histone deacetylases (HDACs) or DNA methyltransferases (DNMTs), resulting in restored melanin production and reduced lipofuscin accumulation [25]. These *in vitro* platforms are becoming essential for testing nutrigenomic and pharmacologic modulators of the pigment epigenome. Compounds like resveratrol, curcumin, and sulforaphane – known to influence chromatin structure – have shown early promise by enhancing melanin synthesis and normalizing pigment granule profiles through targeted epigenetic reprogramming [12, 27].

Moreover, the integration of molecular profiling with high-resolution retinal imaging now enables spatial alignment of pigment anomalies with epigenomic alterations. Techniques such as FAF, near-infrared reflectance (NIR), and melanin-sensitive OCT can noninvasively reveal pigment distribution patterns, which are increasingly being correlated with gene regulatory data from tissue or organoid models. Artificial intelligence (AI)-based analysis of these imaging outputs, when trained on known epigenomic signatures, may facilitate real-time assessment of pigment stability and help predict early risk of degeneration [25, 27, 28]. This synergy between molecular and clinical data forms the basis for identifying at-risk individuals early – while therapeutic modulation of pigmentary balance is still feasible. Encouragingly, longitudinal observations in aging cohorts have demonstrated that pigment gene expression can remain stable – or even be upregulated – in certain elderly individuals with preserved retinal architecture, suggesting the presence of epigenetic resilience mechanisms [25]. The identification of such "epigenetically protected" phenotypes opens new avenues for personalized retinal health strategies, where molecular screening could be used to guide preventive interventions well before the onset of irreversible damage [25, 28]. These advances are consistent with a broader shift in ophthalmic research from reactive treatments to proactive disease interception [27].

As our understanding of pigment regulation in the RPE continues to grow, the possibility of developing targeted, noninvasive therapies aimed at sustaining pigment homeostasis becomes increasingly plausible. Such interventions could involve chromatin-modifying nutraceuticals, imaging-guided therapies, or even AI-supported risk stratification tools, all contributing to early-stage care [25, 27]. Taken together, these findings represent a conceptual shift in how we view pigment metabolism in the retina – from a passive, wear-prone process to a dynamic, epigenetically regulated system. Far from being a static biomarker of aging, pigment granule homeostasis is emerging as a potentially modifiable component of retinal health, supported by a growing body of epigenomic research [25, 26]. This evolving perspective holds promise for the development of predictive biomarkers, earlier diagnostics, and innovative therapeutic strategies to preserve vision as populations age. Continued exploration of pigment regulation through an epigenomic lens is revealing not only pathways of degeneration but also the blueprints for resilience and repair.

2.2 Noninvasive biomarkers for retinal aging: From imaging to epigenetic correlation

Recent findings in noninvasive imaging have made early molecular and subcellular changes detection possible before visible anatomical disruption occurs [21, 22, 27]. Specifically, FAF has proven to be a highly sensitive method of visualizing the autofluorescent properties of bisretinoid-containing lipofuscin granules, offering a powerful marker of intracellular oxidative burden and pigment accumulation [18, 19, 29]. This imaging modality has gained prominence due to its ability to provide functional information about RPE cells, particularly highlighting regions under oxidative stress or those with abnormal metabolic turnover [1, 18, 27].

Oxidative stress arises when there is an imbalance between the generation of ROS and the body's capacity to detoxify these intermediates or repair the resulting damage [12, 13, 17]. Essentially, when cells are exposed to excessive levels of reactive oxygen compounds, they become vulnerable to degradation and dysfunction. ROIs can be classified based on their chemical nature, site of origin, target specificity, and their categorization as either radical or non-radical species. Among the various free radicals found in biological systems, oxygen-derived radicals are the most significant in humans. These include singlet oxygen, hydrogen peroxide, superoxide anion, and hydroxyl radicals. ROS and reactive nitrogen species (RNS) are the two main subgroups of free radicals, with the latter – including nitric oxide, nitrous oxide, peroxynitrite, nitroxyl anion, and peroxynitrous acid – often regarded as a subclass of ROS [2, 25].

FAF is especially valuable because it reflects dynamic changes in RPE health that are otherwise invisible with conventional imaging. Likewise, high-resolution imaging of the retina can be achieved using OCT, which allows clinicians to detect subtle irregularities in RPE reflectivity, early signs of pigment epithelial detachment, or the presence of subretinal fluid [21, 22, 30]. OCT also enables quantitative assessment of retinal layer thickness, identifying incipient thinning of the outer retina that may reflect early degeneration. The advent of enhanced depth imaging (EDI-OCT) and swept-source OCT further allows detailed visualization of the choroid and its interface with the RPE, a region critical to understanding the metabolic exchanges influencing pigment maintenance and degeneration [27, 31].

These changes often precede vision loss. Detecting them before the onset of clinical symptoms offers a significant opportunity for early-stage therapeutic intervention. In fact, longitudinal studies have shown that subtle abnormalities detected via OCT and FAF may serve as early predictors of disease conversion, for instance, from early to intermediate age-related macular degeneration (AMD), underscoring the prognostic value of these modalities [1, 25, 32].

When interpreted together, FAF and OCT can offer a holistic perspective: FAF maps the status of RPE cells from a biochemical standpoint, using lipofuscin signal intensity and spatial distribution, while OCT detects microstructural changes in retinal architecture [22, 29]. Integrating these two tools has been shown to significantly improve diagnostic sensitivity and specificity. Regions of increased FAF often correspond to areas of RPE stress or impending atrophy visible on OCT, creating a multi-layered understanding of disease progression. In particular, the juxtaposition of hyperautofluorescent borders with hypoautofluorescent zones in geographic atrophy is associated with boundary expansion and RPE cell death, as validated in multiple clinical trials [1, 22].

This approach allows clinicians to track the dynamics of metabolism *in vivo*, monitor the progression of subclinical disease, and identify windows for early intervention. Furthermore, advancements in image analysis powered by AI now enable automated quantification of FAF and OCT biomarkers, enhancing reproducibility and reducing interobserver variability [25, 27, 28]. These tools are increasingly being used in both research and clinical settings to develop personalized disease trajectories and risk stratification models. Such technologies have already been incorporated into monitoring protocols for dry AMD and inherited retinal dystrophies [26, 27].

Moreover, studies have demonstrated that increased autofluorescence signal correlates with zones of future RPE degeneration, establishing FAF as a predictive biomarker for pathological progression in AMD and other related disorders [22, 29]. In this context, FAF not only serves as a diagnostic aid but also as a therapeutic biomarker to evaluate the efficacy of interventions aimed at modulating oxidative stress, lipofuscin accumulation, or pigment regulation [12, 18, 27]. Novel compounds targeting the Nrf2 pathway or mitochondrial stability are currently in trials, using FAF endpoints to measure changes in oxidative load (see **Figure 1**) [12, 25].

These techniques create the starting point for personalized monitoring and preventive strategy design, especially when used in conjunction with epigenetic profiling or therapeutic trials aimed at modulating pigment metabolism [9, 13, 27]. In the near future, integration of noninvasive imaging with molecular diagnostics, such as miRNA expression, DNA methylation status, or chromatin accessibility mapping, could yield an unprecedented level of precision in managing retinal pigment disorders [9, 20, 25]. This convergence between molecular data and imaging signals may enable clinicians to intervene during the window of reversibility, before irreversible cellular loss occurs [22, 26].

2.3 Noninvasive interventions for pigment homeostasis in the aging retina

On top of the recent findings mentioned previously, a great area of interest is represented by dietary epigenetic modulators, such as polyphenols (e.g., resveratrol, curcumin) and methyl donors (e.g., folate, choline) [10, 11]. These compounds have shown promise in influencing DNA methylation and histone acetylation pathways, which regulate oxidative stress response and melanogenesis [11, 13, 20].

Resveratrol has been shown to activate the Nrf2/HO-1 antioxidant pathway, enhancing cellular defense and promoting survival under oxidative damage characteristic of AMD [12, 33]. Similarly, curcumin activates SIRT1, a HDAC, promoting autophagy and the clearance of damaged organelles, while also preserving

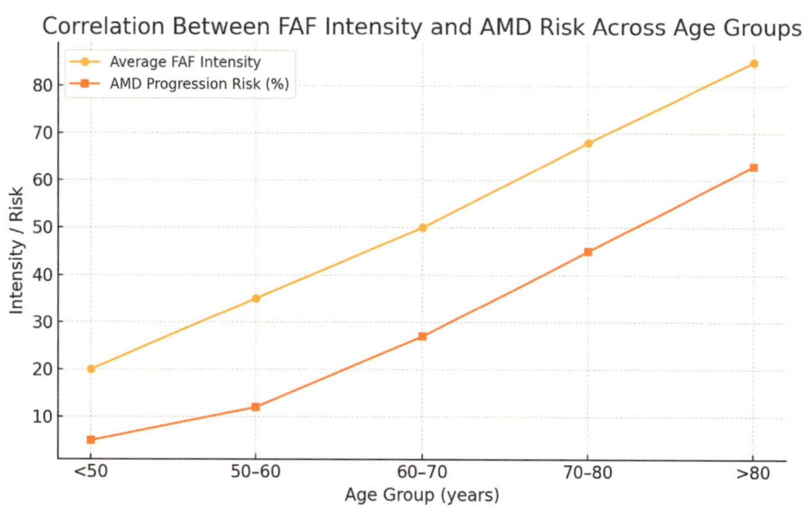

Figure 1.
Correlation between fundus autofluorescence (FAF) intensity and age-related macular degeneration (AMD) progression risk across age groups. Both average FAF intensity (yellow line) and AMD progression risk (orange line) increase progressively with advancing age, with the highest values observed in individuals older than 80 years. Data adapted from the study by Fragiotta et al. [22].

the structural integrity of RPE cells [13, 34]. By contributing to restoring epigenetic homeostasis, these compounds may preserve melanin synthesis and limit the accumulation of oxidative by-products like lipofuscin [18, 33].

In parallel, miRNA-based therapies have proven to be a frontier in modulating gene expression in phagocytic function and RPE pigmentation. Specifically, miR-204/211 are known to influence oxidative defense pathways and melanogenesis [10, 35, 36]. Delivering synthetic mimics or inhibitors via nanoformulation could ultimately lead to targeted control over pigment regulation without affecting photoreceptors or systemic functions.

Worth mentioning are also light-mediated therapies, such as near-infrared light exposure or low-level laser therapy. These are actively investigated for their potential to enhance mitochondrial activity, stabilize intracellular pigment granules, and reduce ROS [14, 25]. Using precisely controlled light wavelengths, these interventions aim to mitigate photo-oxidative stress and extend RPE functional longevity. Such mitochondrial stimulation may help prevent pigment granule destabilization and delay the onset of oxidative degeneration, a process often compounded by mitochondrial DNA damage and reduced repair capacity in aging cells [17, 25]. Clinical trials suggest that specific wavelengths, such as 670 nm, can upregulate anti-apoptotic signaling and mitigate ROS production, improving the viability of RPE cells in aged retinas [14, 25]. The approaches present great potential for preventive application in pre-symptomatic stages, as identified through imaging biomarkers like FAF and OCT [21, 22].

These noninvasive therapies represent a transformative opportunity to shift clinical management from passive monitoring to active intervention, preserving vision by maintaining pigment homeostasis in aging retinal tissues [9, 12, 13]. Rather than relying solely on late-stage symptom detection and damage control, clinicians may soon be equipped to act proactively, targeting the early molecular and cellular disruptions that precede anatomical deterioration. This paradigm shift implies a transition from a reactive to a preventive and precision-based model of care, in which interventions are guided by individualized risk profiles and real-time biological feedback obtained through advanced imaging and molecular diagnostics [22, 25].

The significance of preserving pigment equilibrium, particularly melanin integrity and lipofuscin regulation, extends beyond localized RPE health, as it directly influences the oxidative environment, photoreceptor viability, and overall retinal resilience to age-related degeneration (see **Figure 2**) [1, 2, 18].

Importantly, therapies such as dietary epigenetic modulators, miRNA-based treatments, and light-mediated interventions are not only accessible and well-tolerated but also adaptable to long-term preventive regimens [10, 12, 14]. Their noninvasive nature allows for safe administration across diverse patient populations, including the elderly and those with comorbidities that contraindicate surgical or pharmacological approaches. Furthermore, these strategies open the door to early-stage clinical trials that evaluate functional outcomes and molecular responses before structural changes become irreversible [25, 27].

The integration of these therapeutic modalities with imaging biomarkers – such as FAF and OCT – provides a robust framework for longitudinal monitoring of treatment efficacy and disease progression [27, 29]. Over time, this could reduce the burden of irreversible blindness by intercepting the pathological cascade at its biochemical root. In the broader context of retinal aging, such proactive approaches

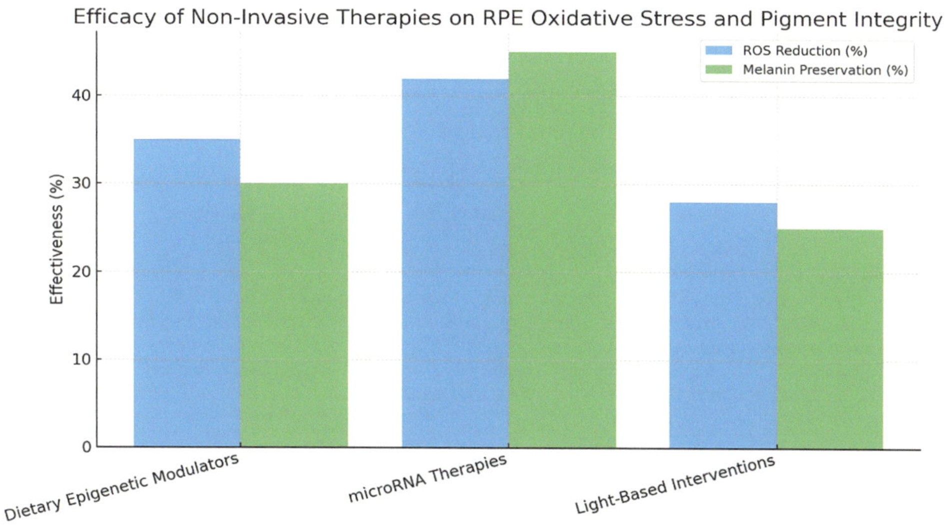

Figure 2.
Efficacy of noninvasive therapeutic strategies on retinal pigment epithelium (RPE) oxidative stress and pigment integrity. Dietary epigenetic modulators, micro-RNA-based therapies, and light-based interventions show variable effectiveness in reducing reactive oxygen species (ROS; blue bars) and preserving melanin levels (green bars). Among these, micro-RNA therapies demonstrate the highest overall efficacy in both ROS reduction and melanin preservation. Data adapted from the studies by Kaur and Elder [27] and Shortt et al. [28].

may redefine the standard of care, focusing on vision preservation rather than delayed symptom management. Ultimately, by maintaining pigment homeostasis through innovative, patient-centered methods, these noninvasive therapies stand to significantly improve quality of life, functional independence, and long-term ocular health for aging individuals worldwide [9, 25, 26].

2.4 A stratified clinical algorithm for the prevention of pigmentary disorders in the aging retina

To operationalize recent scientific advances into clinical workflows, we propose a systematic, evidence-based algorithm designed to prevent pigmentary disorders of the aging retina. This framework integrates deep personalization, epigenetic calibration, and noninvasive monitoring. The overarching objective is to shift the current clinical paradigm from reactive treatment of end-stage pathology to a proactive, stratified model aligned with the principles of predictive and personalized medicine (see **Figure 3** [25]).

Step 1: Identification of risk through multimodal profiling

Comprehensive patient profiling constitutes the initial step in this algorithm. This includes both clinical imaging and molecular biomarker analysis. Clinically, FAF and OCT are already capable of detecting subclinical pigmentary alterations – such as lipofuscin accumulation, melanin depletion, and thinning of the RPE – prior to the onset of symptoms [27].

To complement these imaging modalities, we propose incorporating epigenetic assays using minimally invasive biospecimens (e.g., blood, saliva, tear fluid). These assays would evaluate the methylation status of key

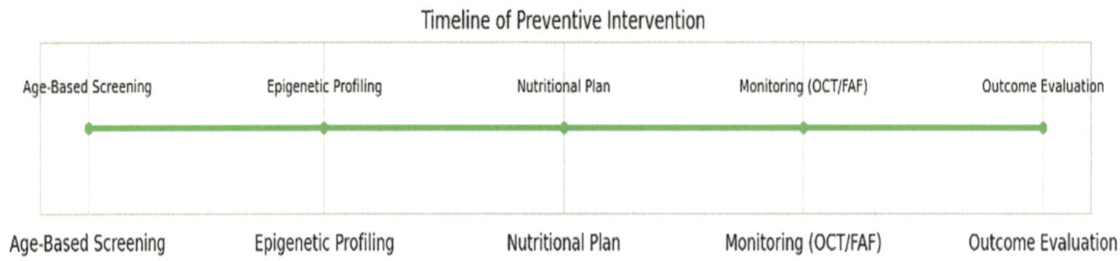

Figure 3.
Timeline of preventive interventions for retinal health. The framework includes sequential steps beginning with age-based screening, followed by epigenetic profiling, implementation of a personalized nutritional plan, longitudinal monitoring using optical coherence tomography (OCT) and fundus autofluorescence (FAF), and final outcome evaluation. This integrative approach emphasizes early detection, individualized prevention, and continuous monitoring to mitigate age-related retinal degeneration.

pigment-regulatory genes (e.g., TYR, OCA2, MITF), histone acetylation levels, and expression patterns of pigmentation-related miRNAs (e.g., miR-204, miR-211) [25, 36]. By integrating molecular and imaging data, patients can be objectively stratified according to their risk of developing pigmentary imbalance and oxidative dysfunction.

Step 2: Stratification into risk tiers

We recommend a three-tiered classification system based on combined clinical and molecular indicators:

Tier I (low risk): Normal FAF and OCT imaging; stable epigenetic profile with no indicators of pigmentary imbalance.

Tier II (moderate risk): Mild anomalies in FAF or OCT reflectivity; evidence of limited epigenetic drift (e.g., minor hypomethylation of pigment-related gene promoters).

Tier III (high risk): Significant imaging abnormalities (e.g., hyper autofluorescence, melanin signal loss, presence of subretinal fluid) coupled with marked epigenetic dysregulation (e.g., repression of miRNAs, global hypomethylation of pigment biosynthesis pathways) [25].

This risk stratification enables the targeted deployment of preventive interventions, optimizing healthcare resource utilization and avoiding overtreatment in low-risk individuals.

Step 3: Implementation of individualized preventive interventions

Preventive protocols are tailored to each risk tier:

Tier III (high risk): Patients will initiate a targeted epigenetic nutritional therapy regimen incorporating resveratrol, curcumin, folate, and choline [25, 31, 32]. Follow-up includes FAF/OCT imaging every three to six months and annual epigenetic profiling to monitor therapeutic response.

Tier II (moderate risk): Patients will undergo a nutritional optimization program emphasizing increased dietary intake of polyphenols (e.g., berries, turmeric, leafy greens) and methyl donors, delivered through dietary counseling. Imaging follow-up is scheduled at 6–12-month intervals, with optional molecular monitoring.

Tier I (low risk): Participants receive general dietary guidance focused on antioxidant-rich nutrition, with annual imaging assessments serving as a baseline comparator for algorithm validation.

Step 4: Adaptive monitoring and dynamic re-stratification

Recognizing the dynamic nature of epigenetic regulation and disease progression, the model incorporates longitudinal follow-up and tier reassignment. Escalation to a higher-risk tier is prompted by worsening imaging features (e.g., increased autofluorescence or pigment epithelial disruption) or molecular indicators (e.g., heightened oxidative stress gene expression, silencing of pigmentary genes). Conversely, sustained structural and molecular stability may justify tier de-escalation, indicating a positive therapeutic response or intrinsic homeostatic resilience [25]. This adaptive feedback loop ensures personalized continuity of care and aligns preventive efforts with each patient's evolving biological profile.

Step 5: Population-level implementation and public health integration

To scale the algorithm for population health, integration with community-based screening programs, electronic medical records (EMRs), and AI-driven decision support systems is essential. Automated FAF/OCT interpretation tools could detect early pigmentary abnormalities, triggering molecular testing and algorithmic risk stratification [27].

Digital platforms may facilitate ongoing engagement by delivering personalized dietary recommendations, appointment reminders, and adherence tracking based on tier status. On a broader scale, public health campaigns could endorse dietary patterns rich in natural epigenetic modulators (e.g., plant-based or Mediterranean diets) to promote retinal health across aging populations [25, 26].

Recent clinical evidence also supports the importance of targeted antioxidant supplementation in maintaining RPE function in aging individuals. In a year-long observational study, patients with age-related maculopathy or diabetic maculopathy received daily doses of dietary supplements, including lutein, zeaxanthin, vitamin E, selenium, and green tea–derived epigallocatechin-3-gallate (EGCG) [34]. The study compared four patient groups – three receiving supplements and one control – and monitored changes using Amsler testing, visual acuity, and fundus ophthalmoscopy.

A supplement, which contains EGCG extracted from *Camellia sinensis*, demonstrated the highest antioxidative capacity *in vitro* (2.778 nmol Trolox equivalents), far exceeding classical lutein-based combinations [34]. Clinically, it showed protective effects on macular function, likely due to its additional properties: upregulation of retinal cell turnover, inhibition of glutamate and nitric oxide neurotoxicity, and improved retinal perfusion. Patients in this group preserved or improved visual function, especially when the EGCG supplement followed prior lutein supplementation [34].

A notable clinical observation found that "after the treatment based on epigallocatechin gallate supplement, some visual parameters improved or at least remained the same compared to the control group without treatment, in which the ophthalmologic situation got worse, more or less" [34]. This strongly supports the potential of natural compounds like EGCG in stabilizing retinal health. Encouraging findings also came from the group receiving the supplement, in the form of overall improvement in retinal health, supported by the increasing cellular turn-over, increased nervous system blood flow, and nourishment of degenerated eye tissues [34].

These findings reinforce the idea that nutritional interventions can stabilize or even enhance pigment homeostasis when applied early and consistently. Furthermore, they underscore the additive value of epigenetically active polyphenols, such as EGCG, in preventive retinal medicine. The synergistic effects of antioxidants, especially those acting through both genomic and epigenetic pathways, provide a strong argument for their integration into early-stage management protocols for pigment imbalance and RPE dysfunction [25, 37].

Another preventive approach is represented by the link between the ocular microbiome and retinal pigmentation. While studies have explored genetic, oxidative, and epigenetic determinants of pigment metabolism, one not fully examined topic is the role of the ocular microbiome, particularly the conjunctival and lacrimal surface flora, in modulating chronic low-grade inflammation and systemic oxidative stress that may affect pigment stability in the RPE [23, 38, 39]. Although anatomically distant, recent evidence suggests a functional axis between the ocular surface and the retina, where immune signals originating from dysbiotic microbial environments on the surface can affect intraocular tissues via circulating cytokines, increased oxidative burden, and modulation of systemic immunity [28, 40].

Especially in aging individuals, the lysosomal degradation pathway can be compromised by this low-grade inflammation, which implies stress on the RPE and accelerates pigment granule imbalance. Chronic dysbiosis has been shown to increase IL-6, TNF-alpha, and NF-κB signaling, which are also upregulated in the degenerating RPE [27, 40].

Beyond inflammation, the microbiome can influence epigenetic processes such as DNA methylation, histone modification, and miRNA expression through microbial metabolites like short-chain fatty acids (SCFAs). These SCFAs, including butyrate and acetate, are known HDAC inhibitors and DNMT modulators, affecting gene expression far from the site of their production [27, 41].

Although most research has focused on the gut–retina axis, ocular-surface-derived SCFAs or immune signals could modulate pigment-related gene expression in the RPE, particularly genes involved in melanogenesis (e.g., TYR, OCA2), oxidative stress (e.g., Nrf2), and phagocytosis (e.g., LAMP2) [18]. Furthermore, miRNAs, such as miR-204 and miR-211, which are crucial in melanin regulation and photoreceptor phagocytosis, may be indirectly regulated by microbial signals. This positions the ocular microbiome as a remote regulator of pigment homeostasis and a potential target for novel therapies [27, 36].

Given the emerging evidence, a new preventive paradigm could include monitoring and modulating the ocular microbiome in aging patients at risk for pigment imbalance. This might involve microbiome profiling tools (e.g., 16S rRNA sequencing from conjunctival swabs) to assess microbial diversity and detect dysbiosis early; topical prebiotics or probiotics formulated to promote beneficial species (e.g., *Staphylococcus epidermidis*, which produces antimicrobial peptides [42, 43]); and anti-inflammatory ocular surface treatments (e.g., omega-3 fatty acids or lactoferrin) to mitigate subclinical inflammation [27].

Integration of microbiome status with FAF/OCT imaging data and epigenomic RPE profiling could support precision prevention. Building upon the expanding field of nutritional epigenetics, experimental studies show the potential of plant-derived antioxidant complexes in preventing maculopathy in aging populations [37, 44]. A surprising result was observed in the usage of a vegetal complex comprised of lutein, zeaxanthin, bilberry extract (*Vaccinium myrtillus*), astaxanthin, zinc, and selenium. This complex was shown to counteract oxidative phototoxicity, inhibit free radical accumulation, and stabilize lysosomal pigment granule turnover [37].

As emphasized in recent analyses, "the retina is particularly susceptible to damage by ROI" [26], a process driven by light exposure, high oxygen consumption, and the presence of photosensitive molecules such as lipofuscin and melanin. ROIs contribute to oxidative stress, damaging RPE cells and destabilizing intracellular pigment granules. Over time, this leads to the hallmark features of retinal aging: lipofuscin accumulation and melanin degradation.

To combat these processes, noninvasive interventions such as antioxidant vegetal supplements have drawn scientific interest. The referenced study evaluated Romanian market supplements used in degenerative ocular conditions, with results supporting their integration into preventive care strategies [45]. A certain vegetal extract, in particular, was identified as the most effective compound tested, with a total antioxidant capacity significantly higher than other formulations – especially due to synergistic ingredients such as homotaurine and *Coleus forskohlii* extract. This points toward a compounded mechanism of protection that includes modulation of oxidative stress and potential epigenetic regulation of pigment maintenance pathways.

Clinically, such antioxidant-rich therapies may help stabilize the oxidative environment of the aging retina, protecting pigment integrity and delaying the onset of anatomical damage. Their ease of administration and favorable safety profiles also make them attractive candidates for early-stage intervention, well before irreversible RPE atrophy occurs.

While oxidative stress is a central component in this cascade, other age-dependent mechanisms, such as mitochondrial dysfunction and lysosomal inefficiency, contribute to pigment instability. The RPE becomes progressively unable to manage the metabolic load, which accelerates pigment granule disruption and drusen formation. Importantly, noninvasive imaging technologies, like FAF and OCT, have enabled early visualization of these subclinical pigmentary changes, allowing for earlier diagnosis and monitoring.

One of the most concerning developments during aging is the accumulation of lipofuscin, a non-degradable pigment granule rich in bisretinoids, known to be phototoxic and pro-oxidative. As the authors of the reviewed study highlight, "Lipofuscin accumulation may, therefore, be the earliest morphological sign of ageing of the retina" [25]. This accumulation not only signals oxidative imbalance but may also contribute to cellular toxicity and inflammation, reinforcing its role as both a marker and a mediator of degeneration.

Preventive strategies aimed at pigment stabilization have begun to emerge, focusing on antioxidant therapy, nutritional modulation, and emerging molecular interventions. Compounds that modulate oxidative stress, such as resveratrol or lutein, and interventions that support lysosomal clearance show potential for clinical translation. As we better understand the epigenetic and metabolic control of pigment homeostasis, targeted noninvasive therapies could delay or even prevent the cascade that leads to RPE dysfunction and vision loss.

A recent study described how the core degenerative pathways of RPE aging directly intersect with these mechanisms, which further promote the value of proper usage of these specific therapies [26]. These antioxidant-rich phytocomplexes could be formally integrated into the Tier II and Tier III prevention protocols outlined in our stratified clinical algorithm. Moreover, they could be used to delay the progression of early pigment imbalance detected via OCT and FAF or as a supportive intervention alongside light-based therapies or miRNA [25, 26].

This integration not only expands the armamentarium of noninvasive prevention tools but also bridges traditional botanical medicine with cutting-edge molecular ophthalmology. Such a multilayered approach could be incorporated into personalized ophthalmic care, where at-risk phenotypes are identified not only through imaging and genetics but also through microbial and epigenetic biomarkers [25]. For instance, patients with reduced microbial diversity, elevated IL-6, and lipofuscin signal on FAF may be stratified into a high-risk group for early intervention [28].

The integration of ocular microbiome science into the field of retinal pigment biology opens new, noninvasive avenues for prevention and early intervention in aging-associated retinal degeneration. While traditionally overlooked, ocular surface health may hold the key to preserving intracellular pigment integrity, not just through barrier function but also via immune and epigenetic signaling [27, 28, 38]. As personalized medicine evolves, including microbiome diagnostics and surface-targeted therapies in the management of retinal health offers a promising frontier to reduce blindness in aging populations – before structural damage begins.

3. Conclusions

As the burden of retinal degenerative disorders continues to rise with global aging, this comprehensive investigation underscores the pivotal role of pigment metabolism within the RPE and the broad spectrum of mechanisms influencing its dysregulation. Through a detailed examination of age-related pigment imbalances, most notably lipofuscin accumulation and melanin degradation, we have revealed the significant contributions of oxidative stress, impaired lysosomal activity, and disrupted intracellular granule turnover as foundational drivers of early RPE dysfunction [44].

This work has explored how advanced imaging modalities, such as FAF and OCT, offer a noninvasive window into detecting biochemical and structural markers of pigment imbalance before irreversible degeneration ensues [25, 27]. These modalities not only serve as predictive biomarkers but also align seamlessly with molecular-level investigations of RPE pathophysiology.

In particular, the central emphasis on epigenetic regulation – through DNA methylation, histone modification, and noncoding RNAs – has opened new frontiers in understanding pigment metabolism as a dynamic and modifiable system. Studies discussed throughout this work have shown that genes associated with melanin synthesis, oxidative defense, and phagocytic activity are tightly regulated by epigenetic cues that deteriorate with age [25, 36]. This degradation, however, is not irreversible, and the exploration of epigenetic plasticity offers tangible therapeutic hope.

One of the key actionable areas identified is the development and implementation of noninvasive strategies rooted in nutritional epigenetics. Bioactive dietary compounds, such as polyphenols (resveratrol, curcumin), methyl donors (folate, choline), and miRNA modulators, have demonstrated the potential to stabilize RPE function by reactivating gene expression programs responsible for pigment homeostasis. Light-mediated interventions further complement these therapies by targeting mitochondrial health and cellular resilience.

Building upon this, we proposed a stratified prevention algorithm based on epigenomic profiling and imaging biomarkers. This model facilitates patient categorization into low-, medium-, and high-risk groups, allowing targeted interventions in alignment with predictive and personalized medicine. When applied early, this strategy may delay or even prevent the onset of advanced retinal pathology [25].

Importantly, this work extended beyond the cellular and molecular lens to include an emerging and largely unexplored factor: the ocular surface microbiome. We have discussed how chronic low-grade inflammation induced by microbiota dysbiosis may indirectly influence pigment metabolism in the RPE, possibly through oxidative pathways and modulation of the host's epigenetic machinery [27, 39].

A growing body of evidence demonstrates that oxidative stress, inflammation, and metabolic dysfunction actively drive pigment imbalance, often preceding anatomical disruption [40, 41, 45]. High-resolution, noninvasive imaging techniques such as FAF and OCT now allow clinicians to detect these early subclinical changes, facilitating prompt interventions [44, 46].

At the cellular level, recent studies emphasize the relevance of RPE detachment, tumor classification, and structural remodeling in visual acuity decline, supporting their role as critical biomarkers of disease progression [44–46]. In parallel, investigations into RPE cell biology and chromatin accessibility reveal that aging-related metabolic reprogramming directly affects pigment granule turnover and melanin preservation [47, 48]. Transcriptomic profiling in geographic atrophy, along with analyses of senescence-related signaling pathways, further clarifies the molecular underpinnings of retinal pigment degradation [49, 50].

Moreover, chronic inflammation and systemic metabolic indicators, such as lipid ratios and neutrophil–lymphocyte imbalances, are increasingly correlated with retinal deterioration and may serve as accessible clinical predictors [42, 43]. Pharmacological therapies that target angiogenesis and lipid metabolism, as well as non-pharmacological options, such as nutritional supplementation with antioxidants and xanthophyll pigments, show promising effects in modulating RPE aging and maintaining retinal integrity [51–57].

Taken together, these insights affirm that pigmentary dysregulation is not only measurable and clinically significant, but potentially modifiable. The future of retinal aging management lies in integrating imaging, molecular diagnostics, and personalized interventions – shifting the paradigm from AMD late-stage treatment to early-stage preservation and prevention [43, 51–55].

The integration of this novel field into the broader understanding of pigmentary regulation introduces compelling research and therapeutic opportunities. Together, these findings present a paradigm shift – from reactive treatment of irreversible degeneration to proactive, multimodal strategies aimed at preserving pigment balance and retinal integrity. The convergence of molecular biology, nutritional science, ocular imaging, and microbiome research fosters a truly interdisciplinary approach capable of reshaping future standards in ophthalmic care. Moreover, the above-mentioned prevention strategies could integrate the similarities between aging pigmentation disorders in both skin and retina, thus creating a new early diagnosis bridge between skin and eye. Therefore, the idea of recommending an ophthalmological examination from the moment of the appearance of aging spots on the skin might be a pertinent suggestion.

This chapter ultimately lays the groundwork for clinical translation, advocating for broader implementation of early screening tools, dietary interventions, epigenetic monitoring, and microbiome research in retinal health. By targeting the earliest molecular vulnerabilities, we may fundamentally alter the trajectory of vision loss in the aging population, transforming pigment regulation from a passive degenerative process into an actively modifiable therapeutic frontier.

Author details

Sanda Jurja[1], Ticuta Negreanu-Pirjol[2,5*], Mihaela Cezarina Mehedinti[3*], Ana Maria Dascalu[4], Florentina Nicoleta Roncea[2], Maria-Andrada Hincu[3] and Bogdan-Stefan Negreanu-Pirjol[2]

1 Faculty of Medicine, Ovidius University of Constanta, University Alley, Constanta, Romania

2 Faculty of Pharmacy, Ovidius University of Constanța, Constanța, Romania

3 Faculty of Medicine, "Dunărea de Jos" University of Galați, Galați, Romania

4 Faculty of Medicine, Carol Davila University of Medicine and Pharmacy, Bucharest, Romania

5 Academy of Romanian Scientists, Bucharest, Romania

*Address all correspondence to: ticuta_np@yahoo.com; mihaela_hincu10 @yahoo.com

IntechOpen

References

[1] Fleckenstein M, Mitchell P, Freund KB, et al. The progression of geographic atrophy secondary to age-related macular degeneration. Ophthalmology. 2018;**125**(3):369–390. DOI: 10.1016/j.ophtha.2017.08.038

[2] Ambati J, Fowler BJ. Mechanisms of age-related macular degeneration. Neuron. 2012;**75**(1):26–39. DOI: 10.1016/j.neuron.2012.06.018

[3] Yiwen Y, Yue W, Leihong X, Picardo M, Chengfeng Z. Deciphering the role of skin aging in pigmentary disorders. Free Radical Biology and Medicine. 2025;**227**:638–655. DOI: 10.1016/j.freeradbiomed.2024.12.032

[4] Hwang ES, Yoon G, Kang HT. A comparative analysis of the cell biology of senescence and aging. Cellular and Molecular Life Sciences. 2009;**66**:2503–2524. DOI: 10.1007/s00018-009-0034-2

[5] König J, Ott C, Hugo M, Jung T, Bulteau AL, Grune T, Höhn A. Mitochondrial contribution to lipofuscin formation. Redox Biology. 2017;**11**:673–681. DOI: 10.1016/j.redox.2017.01.017

[6] Choi SY, Bin BH, Kim W, Lee E, TR L, Cho EG. Exposure of human melanocytes to UVB twice and subsequent incubation leads to cellular senescence and senescence-associated pigmentation through the prolonged p53 expression. Journal of Dermatological Science. 2018;**90**:303–312. DOI: 10.1016/j.jdermsci.2018.02.016

[7] Birch-Machin MA, Bowman A. Oxidative stress and ageing. British Journal of Dermatology. 2016;**175**(2):26–29. DOI: 10.1111/bjd.14906

[8] Gu Y, Han J, Jiang C, Zhang Y. Biomarkers, oxidative stress and autophagy in skin aging. Ageing Research Reviews. 2020;**59**:101036. DOI: 10.1016/j.arr.2020.101036

[9] Grigoryan EN, Markitantova Y. Epigenetic modifications in the retinal pigment epithelium of the eye during RPE-related regeneration or retinal diseases in vertebrates. Biomedicines. 2025;**13**(7):1552. DOI: 10.3390/biomedicines13071552

[10] He L, Hannon GJ. MicroRNAs: Small RNAs with a big role in gene regulation. Nature Reviews Genetics. 2004;**5**(7):522–531. DOI: 10.1038/nrg1379

[11] Martínez-Iglesias ON, Carrera V, Corzo I, Lola Cacabelos R. Natural Bioactive Products as Epigenetic Modulators for Treating Neurodegenerative Disorders. Pharmaceuticals. 2023;**16**(2). DOI: 10.3390/ph16020216

[12] Tahereh F, Folgado SL, Pourbagher-Shahri AM, Ashrafizadeh M, Samarghandian S. The therapeutic effect of resveratrol: Focusing on the Nrf2 signaling pathway. Biomedicine & Pharmacotherapy. 2020;**127**:110234. DOI: 10.1016/j.biopha.2020.110234

[13] Di Gregorio J, Zerti D, Carozza G, Capozzo A, Flati V, Feligioni M, Maccarone R. Hormetic Effects of Curcumin in RPE Cells: SIRT1 and Caspase-3 Inactivation with Implications for AMD. International Journal of Molecular Sciences. 2025;**26**:8555. DOI: 10.3390/ijms26178555

[14] Zadorozhnyy O, Andrii K, Illia N, Taras K, Nevskaya A, Pasyechnikova N. Photobiomodulation therapy in ophthalmology. Oftalmologicheskiĭ Zhurnal. 2022;**100**:47–53. DOI: 10.3128 8/oftalmolzh202254753

[15] Dontsov AE, Ostrovsky M. Retinal pigment epithelium pigment granules: Norms, age relations and pathology. International Journal of Molecular Sciences. 2024;**25**(7):3609. DOI: 10.3390/ijms25073609

[16] Bonilha VL. Age and disease-related structural changes in the retinal pigment epithelium. Clinical Ophthalmology. 2008;**2**(2):413–424. Available from: http s://www.ncbi.nlm.nih.gov/pmc/articles/ PMC2693982/ [Accessed: 2025-June-10]

[17] Wang AL, Lukas TJ, Yuan M, Neufeld AH. Age-related increase in mitochondrial DNA damage and loss of DNA repair capacity in RPE cells. Investigative Ophthalmology & Visual Science. 2008;**49**(4):1801–1807. DOI: 10.1167/iovs.07-1032

[18] Somasundaran S, Constable IJ, Mellough CB, Carvalho LS. Retinal pigment epithelium and age-related macular degeneration: A review of major disease mechanisms. Clinical and Experimental Ophthalmology. 2020;**48** (8):1043–1056. DOI: 10.1111/ceo.13834

[19] Delori FC, Dorey CK, Staurenghi G, Arend O, Goger DG, Weiter JJ. In vivo fluorescence of the ocular fundus exhibits retinal pigment epithelium lipofuscin characteristics. Investigative Ophthalmology & Visual Science. 1995;**36**(3): 718–729

[20] Hushcha Y, Blo I, Oton-Gonzalez L, Mauro GD, Martini F, Tognon M, Mattei MD. microRNAs in the Regulation of Melanogenesis. International Journal of Molecular Sciences. 2021;**22**:6104. DOI: 10.3390/ ijms22116104

[21] Spaide RF, Curcio CA. Anatomical correlates to the bands seen in the outer retina by optical coherence tomography: Literature review and model. Retina. 2011;**31**(8):1609–1619. DOI: 10.1097/ IAE.0b013e3182247535

[22] Ehlers JP, McConville C, Yordi S, Cetin H, Cakir Y, Kalra G, Amine R, Whitney J, Whitmore V, Bonnay M, Reese J, Clark J, Zhu L, Luo D, Jaffe GJ, Srivastava SK. Correlation Between Blue Fundus Autofluorescence and SD-OCT Measurements of Geographic Atrophy in Dry Age-Related Macular degeneration. American Journal of Ophthalmology. 2024;**266**:92–101. DOI: 10.1016/j.ajo.2024.04.031

[23] Ozkan J, Willcox MD. The ocular microbiome: Molecular characterisation of a unique and low microbial environment. Current Eye Research. 2019;**44**(7):685–694. DOI: 10.1080/ 02713683.2019.1575864

[24] Barieva AM, Valiullin VV, Samoilov AN. Changes in the level of tyrosinase expression in the retinal pigment epithelium during the development of experimental optic nerve degeneration. Kazan Medical Journal. 2024;**105**(3):452–458. DOI: 10.17816/KMJ562752

[25] Jurja S, Coman M, Hincu M. The ultraviolet influence upon soft tissues. Romanian Journal Of Morphology & Embriology. 2017;**58** (1):45–52. Available from: https:// www.rjme.ro/RJME/resources/files/ 580117045052.pdf [Accessed: 2025-June-10]

[26] Jurja S, Negreanu-Pirjol T, Roncea F, et al. Anti-aging effect on ocular tissues of antioxidant vegetal supplements from the Romanian market. In: 14th International Multidisciplinary Scientific GeoConference – Surveying Geology & Mining Ecology Management – SGEM 2014; 17-26 June 2014, Albena, Bulgaria. Conference Proceedings, Section Advances in Biotechnology; Vol. **I**, p. 225–230. DOI: 10.5593/sgem2014B61

[27] Tavakoli A, Markoulli M, Papas E, Flanagan J. The Impact of Probiotics and Prebiotics on Dry Eye Disease Signs and Symptoms. Journal of Clinical Medicine. 2022;**11**(16):4889. DOI: 10.3390/jcm11164889

[28] Tîrziu A-T, Susan M, Susan R, Sonia T, Harich OO, Tudora A, Varga N-I, Tiberiu-Liviu D, Avram CR, Boru C, et al. From Gut to Eye: Exploring the Role of Microbiome Imbalance in Ocular Diseases. Journal of Clinical Medicine. 2024;**13**:5611. DOI: 10.3390/jcm13185611

[29] Schmitz-Valckenberg S, Holz FG, Bird AC, Spaide RF. Fundus autofluorescence imaging: Review and perspectives. Retina. 2008;**28**(3): 385–409. DOI: 10.1097/IAE.0b013e318164a907

[30] Keane PA, Sadda SR. Imaging chorioretinal vascular disease. Eye (London). 2010;**24**(3):422–427. DOI: 10.1038/eye.2009.308

[31] Zarbin MA, Casaroli-Marano R, Rosenfeld PJ, et al. Age-related macular degeneration: Clinical findings, histopathology and imaging techniques. Dev Ophthalmol. 2014;**53**:1–32

[32] Cukras C, Wong WT, Caruso R, et al. Longitudinal assessment of visual function and structure in patients with age-related macular degeneration with intermediate disease severity. Ophthalmology. 2010;**117**(12):2500–2510. DOI: 10.1016/j.ophtha.2010.03.058

[33] Lu B, Christensen IT, Ma LW, Yu T, Jiang LF, Wang CX, Feng L, Zhang JS, Yan QC, Wang XL. miR-211 regulates the antioxidant function of lens epithelial cells affected by age-related cataracts. International Journal of Ophthalmology. 2018;**11**(3):349–353. DOI: 10.18240/ijo.2018.03.01

[34] Jurja S, Negreanu-Pîrjol T, Roncea F, et al. Correlation between antioxidant activity of vegetal supplement and age-related maculopathy. In: 14th International Multidisciplinary Scientific GeoConference – Surveying Geology & Mining Ecology Management – SGEM 2014; 17-26 June 2014, Albena, Bulgaria. Conference Proceedings, Section Advances in Biotechnology, p. 321–328. DOI: 10.5593/sgem2014B61/S25.045

[35] Lu LJ, Liu J. Human microbiota and ophthalmic disease. The Yale Journal of Biology and Medicine. 2016;**89**(3):325–330. Available from: https://www.ncbi.nlm.nih.gov/pmc/articles/PMC5001955/ [Accessed: 2025-June-10]

[36] Zegans ME, Van Gelder RN. Considerations in understanding the ocular surface microbiome. American Journal of Ophthalmology. 2014;**158**(3):420–422. DOI: 10.1016/j.ajo.2014.05.008

[37] Doan T, Akileswaran L, Andersen D, et al. Paucibacterial microbiome and resident DNA virome of the healthy conjunctiva. Investigative

Ophthalmology & Visual Science. 2016;**57**(13):5116–5126. DOI: 10.1167/iovs.16-20075

[38] Kugadas A, Gadjeva M. Impact of microbiome on ocular health. The Ocular Surface. 2016;**14**(3):342–349. DOI: 10.1016/j.jtos.2016.01.001

[39] Jurja S, Negreanu-Pîrjol T, Negreanu-Pîrjol B-S, et al. UV radiation influences the total antioxidant capacity of artificial tears (ocular lubricant). In: 16th International Multidisciplinary Scientific GeoConference – SGEM Vienna Green 2016: Nano, Bio and Green – Technologies for a Sustainable Future; 2–5 Nov 2016; Vienna, Austria. Conference Proceedings, Section Advances in Biotechnology, Vol. **III**, p. 395–400. DOI: 10.5593/sgem2016HB63

[40] Negreanu-Pirjol T, Roncea FN, Negreanu-Pirjol BS, et al. Antimicrobial and antioxidant activities of some mouthwashes based on black and red fluid fruits extracts. In: 16th International Multidisciplinary Scientific GeoConference – SGEM Vienna Green 2016: Nano, Bio and Green – Technologies for a Sustainable Future; 2–5 Nov 2016; Vienna, Austria. Conference Proceedings, Section Advances in Biotechnology, Vol. **III**, p. 177–184. DOI: 10.5593/sgem2016HB63

[41] Corradetti G, Karamat A, Srinivas S, Sadda SR. Progression to complete RPE and outer retinal atrophy (cRORA): Post HOC analysis of the GATHER1 trial. Graefe's Archive for Clinical and Experimental Ophthalmology. 2024. DOI: 10.1007/s00417-024-06207-1

[42] Tricorache DF, Dascalu AM, Serboiu C, Bobirca A, Cretoiu D, Bratu D, Tudor C, Tribus LC. The role of inflammation in age-related macular degeneration. Journal of Mind and Medical Sciences. 2023;**10**(2): Article 9. 254–259. DOI: 10.22543/2392-7674.1421

[43] Dascalu AM, Popa Cherecheanu A, Serban D, Alexandrescu C, Stana D, Costea AC, et al. Combined anti-Ang2/Tie and anti-VEGF intravitreal therapy in age-related macular degeneration – A systematic review. Farmacia. 2023;**71**(6):1120–1128. DOI: 10.31925/farmacia.2023.6.2

[44] Makarova MA, Plyukhova AA, Andreeva ES. Influence of Multilayered RPE Detachment on Visual Acuity in AMD. Mod Tech Ophthalmol. 2025;**60**(2):129–130. DOI: 10.25276/2312-4911-2025-2-129-130

[45] Reich E, Thaung C, Sagoo MS. Classification of Retinal and RPE Tumors. In: Singh AD, and Damato, BE, editor 4th Edition. Clinical Ophthalmic Oncology. Springer; 2024. p. 1–4. DOI: 10.1007/978-3-031-72433-6_1

[46] Damato BE. Retinal Pigment Epithelial Lesions. In: Clinical Atlas of Ocular Oncology. Switzerland: Springer Cham; 2022. p. 203–245. DOI: 10.1007/978-3-030-90127-1_6

[47] Wang LC, Cao J, Peng Y, et al. Human Retinal Pigment Epithelium Cells. Cell Proliferation. 2021;**55**(4): e13153. DOI: 10.1111/cpr.13153

[48] Hansman DS, Ma Y, Thomas D, et al. Metabolic reprogramming of the retinal pigment epithelium related macular degeneration. Bioscience Reports. 2024;**44**(4):BSR20231904. DOI: 10.1042/BSR20231904

[49] Senabouth A, Daniszewski M, Lidgerwood, GE, et al. Transcriptomic and proteomic retinal pigment epithelium signatures of age-related macular degeneration. Nature Communications. 2022;**13**:4233. DOI: 10.1038/s41467-022-31707-4

[50] Dhirachaikulpanich D, Lagger C, Chatsirisupachai K, et al. Intercellular communication analysis of the human retinal pigment epithelial and choroidal cells predicts pathways associated with aging, cellular senescence and age-related macular degeneration. Frontiers in Aging Neuroscience. 2022;**14**:1–15. DOI: 10.3389/fnagi.2022.1016293

[51] Dascalu AM, Alexandrescu C, Vancea G, Stana D, Costea DO, Zgura A, et al. The relationship between statin therapy and age-related macular degeneration – A systematic review. Farmacia. 2024;**72**(2):285–293. DOI: 10.31925/farmacia.2024.2.6

[52] Tricorache DF, Dascalu AM, Alexandrescu C, Bobirca A, Grigorescu C, Tudor C, Cristea BM. Correlations between the neutrophil-lymphocyte ratio, platelet-lymphocyte ratio, and serum lipid fractions with neovascular age-related macular degeneration. Cureus. 2024;**16**(6):e62503. DOI: 10.7759/cureus.62503

[53] Vision Loss Expert Group of the Global Burden of Disease Study; GBD 2019 Blindness and Vision Impairment Collaborators. Global estimates on the number of people blind or visually impaired by age-related macular degeneration: A meta-analysis from 2000 to 2020. Eye (London). 2024. DOI: 10.1038/s41433-024-03050-z

[54] Mirescu AE, Deleanu DG, Baltă G, Tofolean IT, Baltă F, Cristescu IE, Jurja S. Retinal vascular diseases highlighted by adaptive optics ophthalmoscopy. Rom J Ophthalmol. 2025;**69**(1). DOI: 10.22336/rjo.2025.07

[55] Jurja S, Negreanu-Pirjol T, Vasile M, Hincu MM, Coviltir V, Negreanu-Pirjol BS. Xanthophyll pigments dietary supplements administration and retinal health in the context of increasing life expectancy trend. Frontiers in Nutrition. 2023;**10**:1226686. DOI: 10.3389/fnut.2023.1226686

[56] Jurja S, Negreanu-Pirjol T, Vasile M, Hincu M, Ciuluvica R, Negreanu-Pirjol B. Comparative antioxidant activity of various ophthalmic product types for artificial tears under different experimental conditions. Experimental and Therapeutic Medicine. 2022;**23**(5):330. DOI: 10.3892/etm.2022.11259

[57] Negreanu-Pirjol B-S, Negreanu-Pirjol T, Busuricu F, Jurja S, Craciunescu O, Oprea O, Motelica L, Oprita EI, Roncea FN. The role of antioxidant plant extracts' composition and encapsulation in dietary supplements and gemmo-derivatives, as safe adjuvants in metabolic and age-related conditions: A review. Pharmaceuticals. 2024;**17**(12):1738. DOI: 10.3390/ph17121738

Chapter 6

Perspective Chapter: Machine Learning Models in Early Diagnosis and Risk Prediction of Skin Cancers

Nina Ivanovic, Marina Adriana Mercioni, Olivia Toma and Raluca Dumache

Abstract

Skin cancer remains one of the most common malignancies worldwide, with early detection and personalised risk stratification being key to improving patient outcomes. In recent years, machine learning (ML) has emerged as a powerful tool in dermatology, offering enhanced diagnostic accuracy, risk prediction, and clinical decision-making as a support for clinicians and patients. This chapter investigates the current and future potential of ML models in the early diagnosis and prognostic modelling of pigmented skin cancers, including melanoma, basal cell carcinoma (BCC), and squamous cell carcinoma (SCC). It examines the evolution of ML architectures, from classical algorithms like support vector machines and random forests to advanced convolutional neural networks (CNNs) and multi-module approaches. Key public datasets such as ISIC and HAM10000 are reviewed alongside their limitations, including the underrepresentation of Fitzpatrick skin types IV–VI. Through comprehensive tables and figures, we synthesise the performance metrics, learning methods, and datasets of leading diagnostic models. Furthermore, we highlight the integration of genomic data, mobile apps, FDA-cleared artificial intelligence (AI) devices, and real-time histopathology tools, as well as the ethical, technological, and regulatory challenges of clinical implementation. Data bias, privacy, and the need for inclusive design to ensure equity across diverse populations will also be discussed. The chapter concludes with a forward-looking perspective on federated learning, augmented reality (AR), and teledermatology (TD), aiming to shape an inclusive and AI-augmented future for skin cancer care.

Keywords: skin cancers, artificial intelligence (AI), machine learning (ML), convolutional neural networks (CNN), dermatology

1. Introduction

Skin cancer remains a significant global public health issue, and its incidence continues to rise across all continents. Non-melanoma skin cancers (NMSCs), such as basal cell carcinoma (BCC) and squamous cell carcinoma (SCC), are the prevalent malignancies encountered in dermatological practice [1, 2]. NMSCs represent over 90% of all skin cancers, while the lethal, continuous melanoma, even if less prevalent, is responsible for the majority of skin cancer-related deaths. According to the World Health Organization (WHO), each year, two to three million NMSCs are diagnosed, and approximately 130,000 new cases of melanomas are uncovered worldwide [3]. Early and accurate diagnosis, particularly of melanomas and other pigmented lesions (BCCs, SCCs), is crucial, as it significantly improves patient prognosis and survival rates [4]. Additionally, clinical and dermoscopic overlaps between benign lesions, such as nevi or seborrheic keratosis (SK), and malignant ones contribute to significant diagnostic uncertainty. Conventional diagnostic methods, which rely on visual inspection, dermoscopy, and histopathological evaluation, have limitations. Due to their time-consuming nature and requirement for expert interpretation, subjectivity, interobserver variability, and potential delays in diagnosis, particularly when faced with atypical presentations, are evoked [5, 6]. Considering these challenges, machine learning (ML), a subset of artificial intelligence (AI), has become a transformative tool in dermatological practice. Convolutional neural networks (CNNs) have demonstrated outstanding performance in analysing dermoscopic and clinical figures. They can provide support in screening, enhance diagnostic accuracy, enable predictive insights, and deliver tailored patient care [7]. One of their key features is their ability to detect subtle morphological features, such as asymmetry, border irregularity, and texture variation, often missed by the human eye [7]. These advanced technologies leverage extensive figure databases and sophisticated computational models to enhance clinical judgment, improve early detection, management outcomes, and metastatic potential across diverse populations [8, 9].

This chapter inspects the transformative potential of AI in the field of dermatology. Furthermore, this medical speciality underscores emerging trends such as federated learning, personalised treatment planning, and the integration of AI with augmented reality (AR) and teledermatology (TD). On a global scale, AI, through its work, highlights its capacity to deliver equitable, efficient, and highly individualised skin cancer care [10, 11]. Systematically, we uniquely aim to synthesise recent developments in ML models and specifically address diagnostic disparities across diverse populations. We review current ML models, the integration of multimodal data, including figures, patient information, and genomics, as well as ethical considerations, along with the implementation barriers related to these technologies [12, 13]. The ethical concerns related to AI integration in dermatology encompass patient privacy, data security, and the potential for AI to substitute human decision-making. Challenges to implementation include the expenses associated with AI systems, the requirement for specialised training, and the reluctance to alter established medical routines [14].

2. Pigmented skin cancer diagnosis: Challenges and diagnostic gaps

Accurate diagnosis of pigmented skin cancers, particularly melanoma, presents significant clinical challenges due to their frequent clinical and dermoscopic overlap with benign pigmented lesions such as melanocytic nevi, SKs, and solar lentigines [15, 16]. Melanomas, especially when pigmented, can closely resemble benign nevi, making early and precise identification more difficult. In contrast, NMSCs, like pigmented BCCs or SCCs, can present atypical patterns, mimicking benign or inflammatory lesions [17].

The clinician's expertise and medical experience lead to diagnostic accuracy. However, even highly skilled dermatologists encounter challenges stemming from variability between observers and the subjective nature of visual assessment [5]. Moreover, variations in speciality training, clinical exposure, and familiarity with diverse lesion presentations lead to inconsistent diagnostic outcomes [6]. Additionally, human diagnostic performance tends to decline with uncommon, unseen during training, and atypical presentations, further exacerbating diagnostic uncertainty [18]. The situation is more pronounced when evaluating amelanotic melanoma or hypopigmented lesions, as these can easily delay early clinical suspicion due to their atypical pigmentation patterns or absence of normal visual features [19].

For instance, amelanotic melanomas or non-melanotic variants of BCCs and SCCs often go unnoticed in the early stages. This can frequently lead to late diagnosis and treatment initiation, which subsequently negatively impacts patient prognosis [20, 21].

These atypical presentations may include lesions that do not follow the typical ABCDE (Asymmetry, Border irregularity, Colour variation, Diameter, Evolution) rule for melanoma, making them more challenging to recognise. The ABCDE rule, for instance, is not present in amelanotic melanomas, and the classical visual appearance of BCCs and SCCs is not present in pigmented BCCs and SCCs. In that sense, clinicians cannot rely on their classical visual criteria to diagnose them. Amelanotic melanomas lack pigment, appearing as an erythematous lesion, which can lead the clinician to consider a more benign or inflammatory condition. Pigmented BCCs and SCCs, on the other hand, can mimic benign lesions like SKs due to their irregular pigmentation pattern [22].

Another common diagnostic deviance occurs with SK, benign pigmented lesions by nature, which exhibit dermoscopic features resembling melanoma or pigmented BCCs [23–25].

Also, melanoma, pigmented BCCs, and SCCs can present themselves under the dermoscope like SK. This mimicking process often appears on elderly or sun-exposed skin, complicating the diagnosis [22, 26, 27].

Table 1 highlights typical and atypical macroscopic and clinical manifestations, including characteristics of pigmented and non-pigmented lesions, whether typical or atypical, and their benign or malignant features.

Region-specific disparities further complicate the scenario. Eastern European populations, for example, experience paradoxically higher melanoma mortality rates relative to incidence. This is indicative of systemic delays in diagnosis, access to specialised care, or gaps in public health awareness campaigns focused on pigmented lesion monitoring [28, 29]. Additionally, global disparities exist regarding Fitzpatrick types IV–VI, whose pigmented lesions manifest differently, necessitating distinct diagnostic criteria and increased clinician awareness to prevent missed or delayed diagnoses [30, 31].

Table 1 highlights the importance of AI integration in dermatology to improve the diagnosis of atypical representations. As shown, the inclusion of SK, malignant mimics, and the atypical representation of these lesions can reduce diagnostic variability. Technological advancements, particularly AI integration, represent promising resources that can enhance clinical diagnostic accuracy, bridge gaps caused by clinician variability, and significantly contribute to an equitable healthcare system [7, 32]. The potential of equitable AI in healthcare relies on accurate diagnosis for every Fitzpatrick type. This contributes to a fairer worldwide

Lesion type	Typical presentation	Atypical presentation	Diagnostic challenge
Basal cell carcinoma (BCC)	Pearly, nodular lesion with telangiectasia. See **Figure 1.**	Pigmented lesion See **Figure 2**	Confused as benign nevus, melanoma, or SK.
Melanoma	Dark, irregularly pigmented lesion (ABCDE rule). See **Figure 3.**	Hypopigmented or amelanotic lesion. See **Figure 4.**	Easily confused with benign or inflammatory lesions.
Squamous cell carcinoma (SCC)	Firm, scaly erythematous plaque; ulcerated lesion. See **Figure 5.**	Pigmented lesion or non-healing inflammatory lesion. See **Figure 6.**	Confused with an inflammatory condition, melanoma, or benign pigmented lesions.
Seborrheic keratosis (SK)	Waxy, stuck-on appearance, pigmented. See **Figure 7.**	Darkly pigmented SK, irritated or inflamed SK, resembling melanoma or pigmented BCC/SCC (irregular pigmentation, pseudo-networks, and globular patterns). See **Figure 8.**	Confused with malignant lesions (Melanoma, pigmented BCCs/SCCs), leading to unnecessary biopsies or delayed diagnosis if malignant.

Table 1.
Typical versus atypical clinical presentation of skin cancer.

healthcare system, fostering trust in the patient–doctor relationship and their perspective on AI integration in dermatology.

3. Current state of ML in dermatology

ML has progressively transformed dermatological practices, evolving significantly over the past two decades. This section provides an overview of the main ML models applied to skin cancer diagnosis, highlighting their input learning methods and diagnostic performances. Historically, dermatology relied on classical ML models, such as support vector machines (SVMs) and random forests. Such systems utilise handcrafted features extracted from figures to differentiate between benign and malignant lesions. These traditional approaches laid the foundation but were limited by their dependency on manually selected features and human-driven feature extraction processes [33]. A pivotal advancement was marked as CNN architectures were able to enhance precision in diagnostic accuracy and expand the potential of ML models within dermatology. CNN architectures automatically learn complex patterns and features directly from unprocessed figure data, significantly surpassing the performance of prior ML models in various studies [34]. Such models have proven themselves in the area of identifying skin lesions, with a diagnostic accuracy that matches or even outperforms experienced dermatologists [7]. Despite ongoing progress, certain challenges persist. CNN architectures require large volumes of accurately labelled figures for training, typically sourced from extensive datasets. The ISIC Archive and HAM10000 are essential for creating and testing those algorithms [8, 9]. However, most of these datasets predominantly include figures of light Fitzpatrick groups (I–III), which can introduce bias and reduce the accuracy of algorithms when applied to individuals with Fitzpatrick

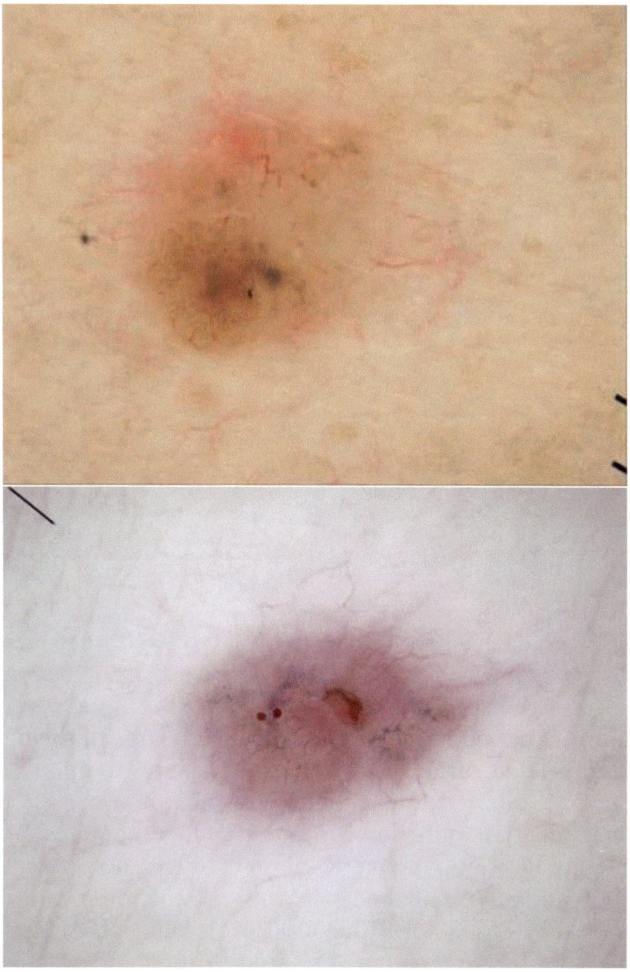

Figure 1.
Dermoscopic figure showing a pigmented skin lesion with an erythematous background, irregular brown pigmentation, and visible superficial telangiectatic vessels. BCCs. [9].

IV–VI [12]. In that sense, to ensure equitable performances across all Fitzpatrick groups, a crucial need for more diverse and inclusive datasets is warranted.

Table 2 provides an overview of the most well-known ML models used extensively in the diagnosis of skin cancer. Each model is summarised with its input type, primary application, learning method, area under the curve (AUC), and the dataset on which its algorithm was trained. This framework demonstrates how to evaluate the diversity of certain datasets, the algorithm type, and how input modality influences performance and output information.

ML models for skin cancer diagnosis have evolved over the past 10 years, with CNN architectures as the dominant algorithm due to their ability to learn multifaceted visual patterns. These architectures are predominantly used on dermoscopic and macroscopic photographs to differentiate certain benign lesions, such as nevi or SK, from malignant ones, such as BCCs, SCCs, or the lethal melanoma. As shown in **Table 2**, CNN architectures such as Inception-v3 [42] and

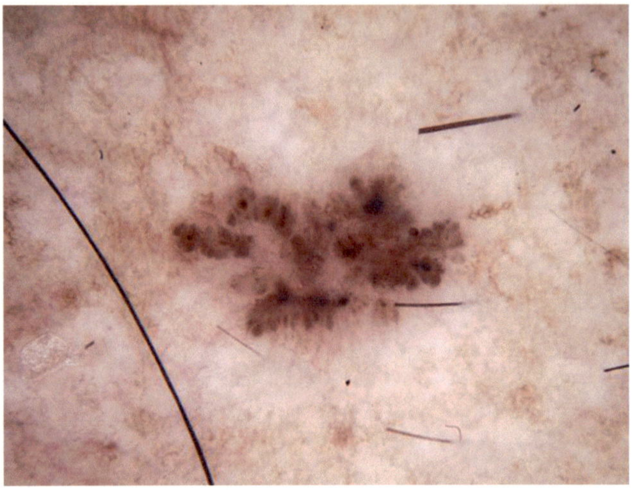

Figure 2.
Dermoscopic figure showing a pigmented skin lesion with irregularly distributed brown globules, heterogeneous pigmentation, and clustered pigmented structures on a light background. BCC [9].

ResNet-50 [34] have achieved an AUC higher than 0.95, trained on the ISIC and HAM0000 datasets. Efficient Net [35] as well is exceeding 0.90 with AUC. These architectures work with processed figure features like asymmetry, border irregularity, colour variation, dimension or diameter, some of them even evolution over a period of time, and surface texture. The concept is to mimic key clinical diagnostic criteria but minimise subjective variability in human judgment [7].

More than classification tools, some ML models incorporate additional data such as patient age, lesion location, or genetic markers to enhance predictive diagnosis. Cutaneous AI [43] and multimodal deep learning (DL) systems were trained on datasets such as PAD-UFES-20 or BCN20000 [44], being able to not only identify malignant skin lesions but also support risk stratification and provide a personalised decision for the patient. Some of these technologies include generative adversarial networks (GANs) like DCGAN and CycleGAN [45], which are able to generate synthetic figures and train simultaneously the generator and the discriminator. Studies have shown that this particular architecture is useful for better exemplifying Fitzpatrick IV–VI skin types or atypical or underrepresented skin lesions. Additionally, federated learning is being explored to allow model training across multiple institutions while preserving patient data privacy, an important key to data sharing and diversity in the datasets [10].

However, as **Table 2** highlights, many of these datasets overrepresent Fitzpatrick I–III types, raising concerns about their accuracy for diverse populations (see Section 7).

Recent progress in various imaging techniques, such as standard clinical photos, dermoscopy, confocal microscopy, and three-dimensional (3D) whole-body scans, has expanded the data sources available for ML models. These techniques bring richer information to the models, helping detect subtle diagnostic prompts that might be missed during standard visual assessments [46].

Addressing existing data constraints and enhancing imaging consistency are crucial for future advancements. By emphasising datasets with diverse, balanced, and standardised figures, ML models will improve their robustness and reliability in advancing skin cancer diagnosis and treatment globally.

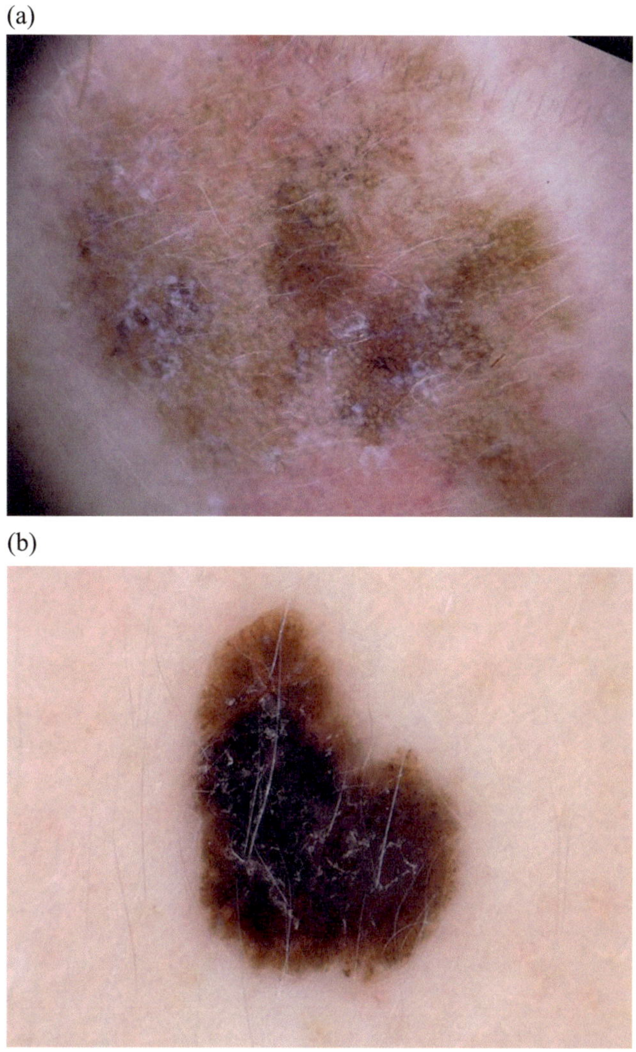

Figure 3.
(a) Dermoscopic figure showing a pigmented skin lesion with heterogeneous pigmentation, multiple irregularly distributed brown areas, colour variation from light to dark brown, whitish scar-like areas, and uneven structural patterns on a pinkish background. Melanoma. [9]. (b) Dermoscopic figure of a pigmented skin lesion with an asymmetric shape, irregular borders, and marked colour heterogeneity, including dark brown to back areas. Melanoma.

4. ML models for diagnosis of pigmented lesions

ML models have been developed extensively to classify skin lesions as malignant or benign, frequently achieving diagnostic accuracy comparable to that of experienced dermatologists in controlled studies. Deep CNN architectures have demonstrated remarkable capabilities by automatically identifying subtle patterns of asymmetry, border irregularities, colour variation, and texture changes correlated with malignancy [47].

Melanoma's criteria versus nevus classifications in CNNs' architectures have tremendously shown high sensitivity and specificity. Studies have demonstrated that

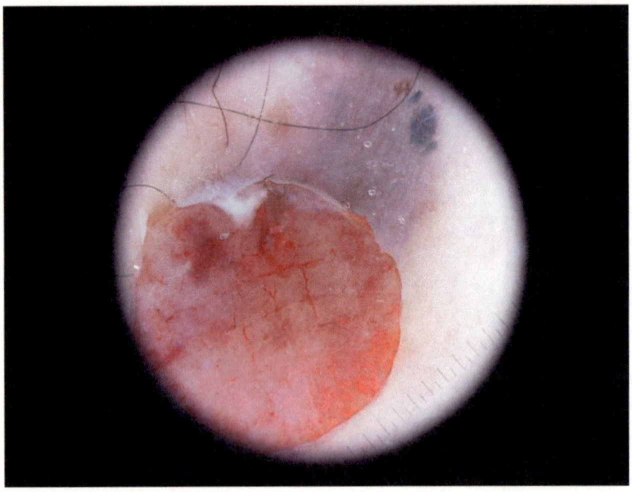

Figure 4.
Dermoscopic figure showing a pink to reddish skin lesion with a relatively symmetric round shape, regular borders, and visible superficial vascular structures and focal hemorrhagic areas. Atypical Melanoma.

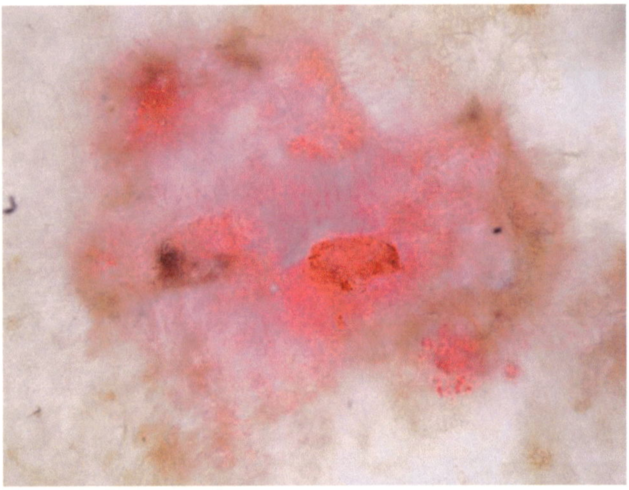

Figure 5.
Dermoscopic figure showing an irregular pink to reddish skin lesion with poorly defined borders, heterogeneous colouration, erosive and crusted areas, and focal superficial hemorrhagic zones. SCC. [9].

CNNs' architectures were matching or even surpassing human experts in this field of diagnosis. Effectiveness is typically assessed using metrics like area under the curve (AUC). Recent research reports CNNs achieving AUCs above 0.90, sensitivity around 90%–95%, and specificity frequently exceeding 85% [7, 32].

Apart from melanoma, AI integration has been effective in distinguishing other pigmented cancers, such as pigmented BCC or SCC, from benign lesions that resemble SKs or inflammatory conditions. By analysing subtle morphological patterns that may not be easily noticeable to human observers, these models were able to reduce diagnostic uncertainty and variability [48].

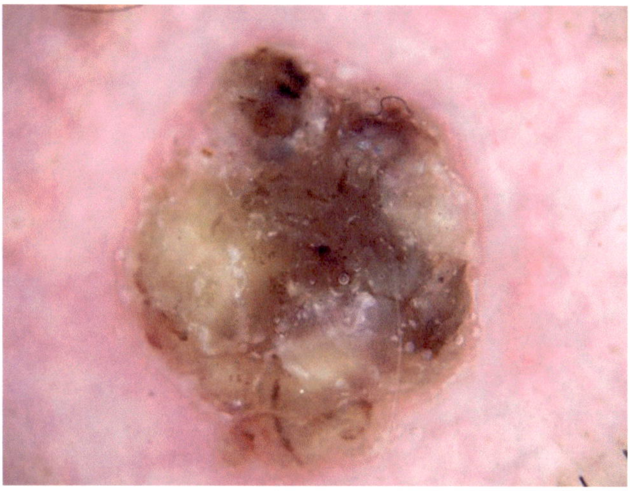

Figure 6.
Dermoscopic figure showing an irregular pink skin lesion with unevenly distributed yellowish to whitish keratinous areas, scattered brownish hemorrhagic zones, scaling and crusts, heterogeneous colouration, and poorly defined borders. SCC. [9].

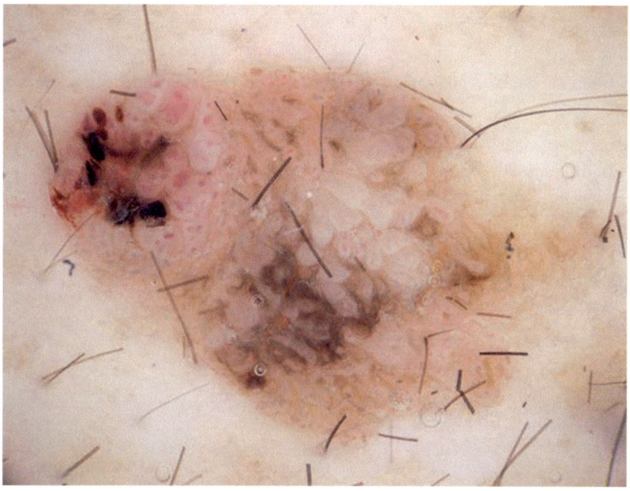

Figure 7.
Dermoscopic figure showing a well-circumscribed brown skin lesion with heterogeneous brown pigmentation, multiple rounded keratinous and papular surface structures, whitish areas, and focal brownish to reddish hemorrhagic zones on a lightly pigmented background skin. SK. [9].

Brinker et al. [34], in their recent study, highlighted a case where an AI system identified an amelanotic melanoma at an early stage. Clinically, the patient presented with a hypopigmented lesion, which was initially diagnosed as benign through dermoscopy. Moreover, this algorithm was able to provide a high malignancy probability score, leading to a biopsy excision where malignancy was confirmed by histopathology [34].

Despite these promising outcomes, significant limitations remain. The first limitation is a lack of generalisability when applied to figures outside the specific training set. Many models' algorithms then exhibit decreased accuracy across

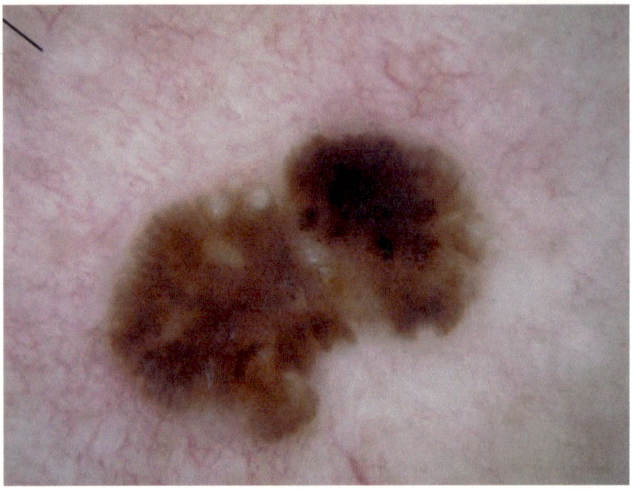

Figure 8.
Dermoscopic figure showing a well-defined brown skin lesion with heterogeneous light to dark brown pigmentation, multiple rounded and lobulated pigmented areas, cerebriform surface structures, and focal whitish keratinous zones on a lightly pigmented background skin. Atypical SK. [9].

Model name	Input type	Application	Method of learning	Reported accuracy/ AUC	Datasets used	Reference
Inception-v3 CNN	Dermoscopy/ Clinical figures	Melanoma classification	Supervised deep learning (CNN)	AUC 0.96	ISIC archive	[7]
ResNet	Dermoscopy/ Clinical figures	Skin lesion classification	Supervised deep learning (ResNet)	AUC 0.95	HAM10000, ISIC2018	[34]
Efficient Net	Dermoscopy figures	Skin lesion classification	Supervised deep learning (EfficientNet)	Top-1 Acc ~89%	ISIC archive, BCN20000	[35]
MobilenetV2	Smartphone figures	Mobile based screening	Supervised deep learning (lightweight CNN)	AUC 0.88–0.90	ISIC archive, PAD-UFES -20	[32]
Random forest	Handcrafted features	Lesion type classification	Supervised machine learning	Acc ~85%	PH2 dataset, DermIS	[36]
Support vector machine	Handcrafted features	Melanoma versus benign classification	Supervised machine learning	Acc ~82-86%	PH2, Derm7pt	[37]
Multimodal CNN (Figure + Metatadata)	Figures + Clinical metadata	Risk prediction/ stratification	Multimodal deep learning	AUC ~0.91; Sens ~87%	ISIC + Custom clinical metadata	[38]
Histopathology CNN (e.g., Clam)	Whole slide figures	Tumour grading/ prognostics	Supervised deep learning (Histopath. CNN)	AUC >0.90 for metastasis prediction	TCGA, private WSIs	[39]

Model name	Input type	Application	Method of learning	Reported accuracy/ AUC	Datasets used	Reference
Vision transformers	Skin figures	Emerging for lesion classification	Transformer-based deep learning	AUC ~0.90	ISIC 2020, FigureNet	[40]
GANS	Synthetic data generation	Data augmentation only	Unsupervised/ generative learning	Synthetic data use only; improves model training	ISIC, generated via DCGAN/ CycleGAN	[41]
Federated learning dermatology AI	Distributed private figure data	Cross-centre diagnosis without sharing data	Federated deep learning	Comparable AUC to centralised models	Federated ISIC dataset subsets, institutional data	[10]

Table 2.
Summary of key machine learning models for skin cancer diagnosis.

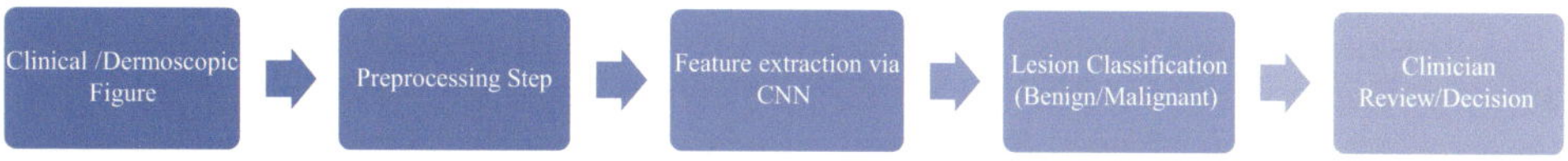
Clinical /Dermoscopic Figure
Preprocessing Step
Feature extraction via CNN
Lesion Classification (Benign/Malignant)
Clinician Review/Decision

Figure 9.
Workflow of a CNN architecture for skin lesion classification. Adapted from the general methodology in the studies by Esteva et al. [7] and Tschandl et al. [32]. Flowchart illustrating a convolutional neural network workflow for skin lesion analusis, showing a sequence from clinical or dermoscopic figure input, preprocessing, feature extraction using a CNN, lesion classification into benign or malignant categories, and final clinician review and decision.

diverse populations or imaging sources. Moreover, data bias is particularly problematic, as most training datasets disproportionately represent lighter skin types, with notable underrepresentation of Fitzpatrick IV–VI types. Additionally, these algorithms have imbalanced datasets, which reduces their performance and accuracy when diagnosing lesions in individuals with Fitzpatrick IV–VI. Such limitations can potentially perpetuate existing healthcare disparities [12, 49].

New strategies should be explored, including data augmentation, federated learning, and domain adaptation. The aim would be to reach a fairer and more robust algorithm [10, 12].

A workflow for CNN architecture is provided in **Figure 9**. This schematic representation highlights the classical CNN architectures. On one hand, the input, dermoscopic figure, and the output, which includes lesion classification as benign or malignant, along with clinician review. This continuous flow emphasises AI integration in dermatology with real clinical decision-making.

Addressing these limitations requires systematic improvements, such as the collection of more diverse, representative datasets and rigorous validation across varied demographic groups. Nevertheless, when deployed responsibly and alongside clinical judgment, ML models serve as valuable adjunctive tools, enhancing early detection and reducing human diagnostic error in dermatology practice.

5. Risk prediction and prognostic modelling

Far from merely identifying a lesion as malignant, AI models predict the risk and provide prognostic outcomes for skin cancer. Thus, ML models integrate dermoscopic and histopathological metadata to forecast aggressiveness, responses, metastatic behaviours, and recurrence risk. For instance, AI applied to microscopic slides of skin tumours predicts metastasis or recurrence by analysing tumour architecture and immune cell infiltration patterns that may elude human perception [39].

Additionally, comprehensive ML approaches that combine clinical parameters, such as patient age, lesion characteristics, and genetic markers, have demonstrated better outcomes than traditional risk assessment frameworks. Recent studies using this model have identified novel risk factors, which are significantly enhancing patient prognostics in skin cancer [50]. Regarding genetic markers in dermatology, mutations in BRAF, NRAS, and KIT from patients have been introduced into ML models. These models, called patient-specific AI integration, can personalise the input, leading to outputs that are more specific to a patient. The particularity resides even in asymptomatic stages, providing them with a personalised therapeutic option for skin cancer treatment [51, 52].

In melanoma specifically, ML models, by predicting recurrence and the necessity of adjuvant therapy, are assisting personalised treatment strategies and optimised follow-up protocols [4, 53]. These tools support clinical decisions made by dermatologists, but they also play a role in adjusting the follow-up intensity and treatment possibilities for each patient. **Figure 10** illustrates how Pluridata inputs are integrated into an AI system to assist clinicians in classifying and predicting risk for patients, offering a personalised approach tailored to each individual's background.

Despite these advancements, limitations persist, notably the requirement for large-scale, diverse, and well-validated outcome datasets before clinical implementation becomes widespread. Nevertheless, ML prognostic models offer promising tools to guide personalised clinical management and preventive strategies, contributing significantly to improved patient outcomes.

6. Innovative applications and recent advances

To successfully benefit patients, AI integration tools must be flawlessly incorporated into clinical practice and the diagnostic workflow. The current applications used in clinical practice range from a variety of smartphone screening apps to FDA-approved devices and high-level AI-integrated microscopes.

Skin Vision uses smartphone technology and AI algorithms to allow users to screen skin lesions. This concept was trained with DL models to analyse uploaded figures and provide risk assessments. Of course, the application was provided as the first step in identifying suspicious lesions. Unfortunately, the application's reliability varies a lot, despite its accessibility and potential for early lesion detection. Thorough validation and regulation policies are needed [54].

At a more advanced and regulated level, wearable diagnostic devices have emerged, such as the FDA-cleared DermaSensor. This handheld, AI-driven device utilises near-infrared (NIR) spectroscopy combined with ML models to non-invasively detect melanoma, BCC, and SCC. Clinical studies indicate that DermaSensor achieves approximately 96% sensitivity, significantly reducing missed cancer cases in clinical settings [55].

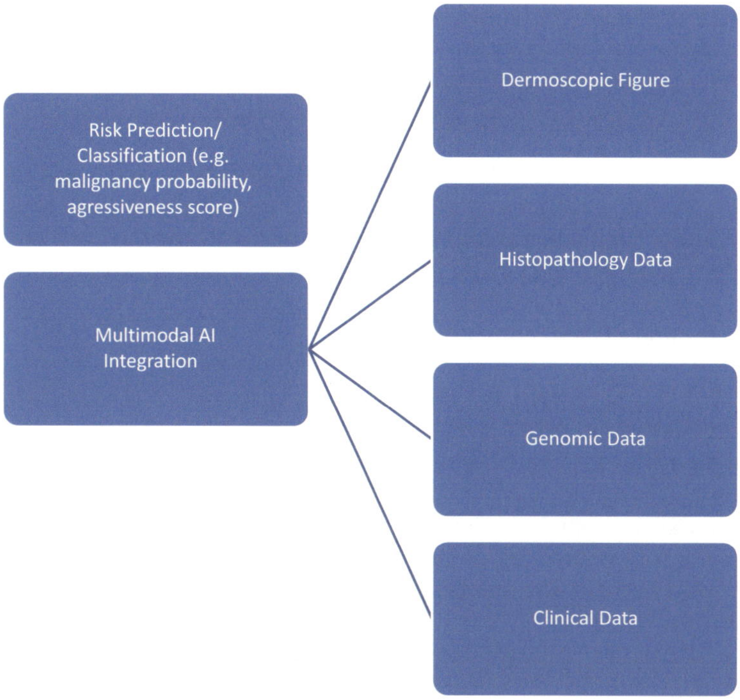

Figure 10.
Multimodal data integration for AI-based diagnostic modelling. Conceptual diagram inspired by Sheller et al. [10], Lu and Mahmood [39], and Liu et al. [50]. Conceptual diagram illustrating multimodal AI integration for skin cancer modelling, with dermoscopic figures, histopathology data, genomic data, and clinical data converging into a central multimodal AI system, which outputs risk prediction and classification measures such as malignancy probability or agressiveness score.

AI integration in microscopy has also demonstrated considerable improvements in real-time histopathological analysis. Such microscopes, powered by AI, enable pathologists to rapidly identify subtle morphological patterns indicative of malignancy. Thereby, diagnostic accuracy, efficiency, and consistency in skin cancer evaluations are improved [56]. Moreover, the integration of NIR spectroscopy with ML models has materialised as an innovative diagnostic approach. NIR spectroscopy non-invasively characterises biochemical properties of skin tissues, and, with ML models, interprets spectral data. Its accuracy in distinguishing malignant from benign lesions provides a fast diagnosis without the need for invasive procedures such as skin biopsy [57].

Several worldwide and multidisciplinary collaborations related to AI have taken place. Google's AI research team has agreed to test a large-scale mobile screening platform with the help of Stanford and Indian dermatology networks. Their work particularly targeted underserved regions, such as rural areas in India [58]. In Europe, the project iToBoS is developing a full-body 3D skin analysis with AI across centres [59]. These studies highlight a worldwide trend in the clinical adoption of AI, while also illustrating AI's potential in both advanced and resource-limited settings.

These AI tools, while promising, require careful integration into existing clinical practices. Criteria such as interpretability, data privacy, and regulatory compliance must not be overlooked. A need for validation and continuous improvement is also essential to fully integrate ML models as assistants in dermatology practice.

Moreover, understanding the patient's point of view on AI remains essential. Recent studies show that some patients value AI-diagnosis for its speed and accuracy, but others remain vocal about their concerns regarding trust and the idea of depersonalisation through this method. Honest communication and integrating the patient into the management of decision-making regarding their skin, their pathology, and a clinician as a mediator between AI and the patient's concerns should help regain confidence and acceptance in the tool [60, 61].

7. Challenges and ethical considerations

While **Table 2** highlights the diagnostic performance of leading ML models in skin cancer detection, it also identifies some limitations that need to be addressed critically to ensure ethical and equitable AI integration in dermatology. A striking issue is that most high-performing algorithms rely on large public datasets, such as the ISIC Archive and HAM10000 [8, 9, 35], which are predominantly composed of light Fitzpatrick skin figures (Fitzpatrick types I–III) [12]. As a result, the models are strictly trained on Fitzpatrick I–III, excluding individuals with Fitzpatrick IV–VI, and potentially perpetuating healthcare disparities through diagnostic inaccuracies.

The use of AI in skin cancer treatment raises critical ethical questions. Concerns about data bias and significant practical challenges must be cautiously managed to ensure fairness, safety, and effective healthcare services for all patient groups.

Current AI algorithms learn from data involving lesions on lighter Fitzpatrick skin types. In this framework, the ethical concerns orbit around the representability of all Fitzpatrick skin types in the dataset. Indeed, such algorithms, when trained on these datasets, compromise diagnostic precision for individuals with Fitzpatrick IV–VI. Healthcare inequalities are exacerbated by these disparities and, moreover, cause inaccuracies with or underdiagnosed lesions for marginalised populations [12]. In addition, demographic factors such as patient age, sex, and lesion location have been shown by Winkler et al. [62] in their study. They were able to demonstrate how sensitivity varies significantly across subgroups, meaning that these demographic factors influence AI diagnostic performance [62].

To minimise this bias, dedicated efforts should aim at enhancing diversity in training datasets. Synthetic data generation and federated learning are able to collect data from multiple centres while also protecting patient privacy and ensuring ethical management. This represents a crucial aspect, especially considering the sensitive nature of dermatological figures and patient information used in AI training and deployment. Some essential traits, such as compliance with strict privacy laws and transparent data handling, are required to instil trust in the patient's perspective and among healthcare providers. Implementing ethical AI involves obtaining clear patient consent, explaining data usage transparently, and applying strong safeguards against misuse or unauthorised access [13].

Other challenges, such as the clinical and technological implementation of these tools, are hindering AI integration in the medical system. In the clinical setting, practitioners must understand the AI-generated recommendations to be able to integrate the information into a strategic patient treatment plan [63]. Moreover, some frameworks should be developed to help AI tools deploy safely and efficiently. On a technological level, these algorithms require specific data formats, high-quality picture resolution, and sufficient computing resources and storage. It is also important to address that these particular requirements are insurmountable barriers for resource-limited hospitals, such as those in lower-income countries [64].

To overcome these biases, the future new models or algorithms should prioritise more diverse input photographs or information. Also, strategies including synthetic augmentation, such as GANs and federated learning in the models [10], can ensure robust performance across all Fitzpatrick skin types and demographic groups. In other terms, GANs could generate lesions and figures on Fitzpatrick IV–VI.

Additionally, AUC scores greater than 0.90, considered a good metric, are often observed in datasets with ideal conditions. On the ground, these metrics/results can deteriorate due to variability in figure quality, device differences, clinical environments, and improper device use. Performance degrades, and thus AUC scores are affected. In this sense, to bridge the gap between ideal conditions in research and real-life practice, rigorous multicentre validation and continuous post-deployment monitoring are essential [34].

The current success of AI in clinical settings relies on regulatory frameworks. The FDA and EMA have created preliminary regulations for AI and medical devices. STARD-AI guidelines, as a dermatology evaluation protocol, are essential to implement assessment and ensure safety and fairness around these tools [65, 66].

Furthermore, multi-speciality teams are required, such as dermatologists, histopathologists, data experts, ethicists, regulators, and patient groups, to address and work on implementing those challenges. If the ethical regulations, data biases, and technological challenges are effectively addressed, AI algorithms and their powerful capabilities could benefit not only dermatologists in their clinical practice but also provide fairer care for patients worldwide.

8. Future directions and innovations

The future directions in this field reside in offering a more personalised, accurate, and accessible strategy to detect and predict skin cancer. AI algorithms represent the future of dermatology. Emerging trends, such as federated learning, propose cutting-edge solutions for adopting data security and privacy measures. Additionally, the desire to train an AI algorithm using data from multiple institutions around the world, without sharing sensitive patient-related information – thanks to federated learning – can expand the diversity of the datasets, enhancing AI diagnostic performance across various Fitzpatrick groups as well as genomic and ethnic backgrounds [10].

Personalised medicine in dermatology can be profoundly augmented by AI. By combining clinical figures, histopathological data, genomic information, and real-time patient monitoring, the goal of "personalised medicine" can be achieved. AI-driven personalised treatment plans will allow for more tailored therapeutic approaches, effectively predicting disease progression, recurrence, and patient response to treatments. Furthermore, continuous patient monitoring through AI-powered wearable technologies will offer unique capabilities for longitudinal tracking of skin lesions, swiftly alerting patients and clinicians to significant changes and enabling timely interventions [67].

Another emerging frontier is AR and TD, capable of enhancing real-time diagnostics remotely. AR platforms would be used to visualise AI-generated perceptions directly on the patient's skin. This will optimise the assessment of the lesion and inform the decision regarding follow-up, treatment, and more broadly, the decision-making process. Additionally, teledermatology platforms enriched with AI models will democratise specialised dermatological care, reaching remote and underserved communities, thereby significantly reducing disparities in skin cancer outcomes worldwide [11].

AI's true potential extends beyond being merely a diagnostic tool; it acts as a valuable partner that enhances human clinical judgment and decision-making. Future AI algorithms should emphasise interpretability and transparency to build trust among clinicians and patients. By combining advanced AI technologies and healthcare methods, alongside dermatologists, a new era of enhanced precision, greater accessibility, and equity in global skin cancer care is created.

MelaFind represents a dermatology AI device that was approved by the Food and Drug Administration (FDA) in 2017. This device was used; however, due to its low specificity (10%), which led to an increased number of unnecessary biopsies [68], the AI device was retracted from the market. Another AI device authorised by the FDA in 2017 for use in dermatology for melanoma diagnosis was Nevisense, with a sensitivity of 96% and a specificity of 34%. This AI device remained on the market until 2024 [69].

FDA authorised, in January 2024, the first AI medical device to be used in the primary care setting for the detection of skin cancers [70]. The novelty of the device lies in the fact that it is considered the first AI-enabled dermatologic device intended to be used by non-specialists [71].

9. Conclusions

ML algorithms exhibit prodigious potential in improving early detection and risk assessment of skin cancers. In this chapter, we examined how AI models differentiate between malignant and benign lesions, estimate tumour aggressiveness, and help dermatologists make better decisions. Integrating AI into dermatology marks significant progress in medicine. ML tools have already enhanced diagnostic accuracy, prognostic predictions, and personalised treatments, significantly reducing errors and variability caused by human judgment and training.

These tools are designed to be valuable helpers, supporting rather than replacing clinicians' judgment, and enhancing accuracy and efficiency in skin cancer management. To fully realise this potential, collaboration across dermatologists, data scientists, regulators, and ethicists is needed to improve algorithms, conduct exhaustive evaluations, and implement AI safely and fairly. The focus should be on reducing biases to ensure consistent performance across all Fitzpatrick skin types and populations while maintaining a patient-focused approach. In short, AI tools, when carefully designed and used, can greatly enhance our ability to fight skin cancer by facilitating earlier detection and personalised risk assessments. Combining technological advances with clinical expertise and fairness efforts will help build a future where AI assists in saving lives through early detection and better prognostic insights. Future advances like federated learning, personalised medicine, and combining AI with AR and TD are anticipated to increase diagnostic and prognostic accuracy and cumulatively improve healthcare access.

Ultimately, this new AI-driven era in dermatology aims to improve patient outcomes worldwide by addressing disparities and strengthening our fight against skin cancer.

Looking ahead, the future of AI in dermatology lies not only in technological advancements but also in the equity and equitable transformation of the technology. Such a broad AI model regarding skin cancer care is merely going to depend on worldwide and multidisciplinary collaboration, diverse Fitzpatrick representation, as well as diverse skin lesions across the datasets. The aim is to build a tool that not only performs with high accuracy but also addresses underserved regions where diagnostic delays cost lives. With good ethical prudence, a patient-centred design, and strategic assets, AI can become a force, reducing the global burden of skin cancer on patients and on the minds of clinicians, empowering those who treat by bringing trustworthy, timely, personalised care to every skin, everywhere.

Conflict of Interest

The authors declare no conflict of interest.

Author details

Nina Ivanovic[1,2,3,5], Marina Adriana Mercioni[6], Olivia Toma[2,3] and Raluca Dumache[1,4]*

1 Center for Research on the Ethics of Genetic Identification (EtIGen), Victor Babeş University of Medicine and Pharmacy, Timişoara, Romania

2 Morphological Skin Research Center (Morphoderm), Victor Babeş University of Medicine and Pharmacy, Timişoara, Romania

3 Department of Dermatology, Victor Babeş University of Medicine and Pharmacy, Timişoara, Romania

4 Department of Forensic Medicine, Bioethics, Medical Ethics and Medical Law, Victor Babeş University of Medicine and Pharmacy, Timişoara, Romania

5 Doctoral School of Medicine, Victor Babeş University of Medicine and Pharmacy, Timişoara, Romania

6 Victor Babeş University of Medicine and Pharmacy Timişoara, Politehnica University Timişoara, Timişoara, Romania

*Address all correspondence to: raluca.dumache@umft.ro

References

[1] Bray F, Ferlay J, Soerjomataram I, et al. Global cancer statistics 2018: GLOBOCAN estimates of incidence and mortality worldwide for 36 cancers in 185 countries. CA: A Cancer Journal for Clinicians 2018;**68**:394–424

[2] Leiter U, Keim U, Garbe C. Epidemiology of skin cancer: Update 2019. Advances in Experimental Medicine and Biology. 2020;**1268**:123–139

[3] World Health Organization. Ultraviolet (UV) radiation and skin cancer. 2017. Available from: www.who.int/news-room/questions-and-answers/item/radiation-ultraviolet-(uv)-radiation-and-skin-cancer [Accessed: 2025-July-20]

[4] Gershenwald JE, Scolyer RA. Melanoma staging: American Joint Committee on Cancer (AJCC) 8th edition and beyond. Annals of Surgical Oncology. 2018;**25**(8):2105–2110

[5] Elmore JG, Barnhill RL, Elder DE, et al. Pathologists' diagnosis of invasive melanoma and melanocytic proliferations: Observer accuracy and reproducibility study. BMJ. 2017;**357**: j2813

[6] Argenziano G, Cerroni L, Zalaudek I, et al. Accuracy in melanoma detection: A 10-year multicenter survey. Journal of the American Academy of Dermatology. 2012;**67**:54–59

[7] Esteva A, Kuprel B, Novoa RA, et al. Dermatologist-level classification of skin cancer with deep neural networks. Nature. 2017;**542**:115–118

[8] Codella NCF, Rotemberg V, Tschandl P, et al. Skin lesion analysis toward melanoma detection: A challenge at the 2017 international symposium on biomedical imaging. IEEE Int Symp Biomed Imaging. 2018;**2018**:168–172

[9] Tschandl P, Rosendahl C, Kittler H. The HAM10000 dataset, a large collection of multi-source dermatoscopic images of common pigmented skin lesions. Scientific Data. 2018;**5**:180161

[10] Sheller MJ, Reina GA, Edwards B, et al. Federated learning in medicine: Facilitating multi-institutional collaborations without sharing patient data. Scientific Reports. 2020;**10**:12598

[11] Meghe SR, Ramapure R, Singh A, Jawade S. Augmented/virtual reality in dermatology: A digital arsenal in modern era. Journal of Pharmacy and Bioallied Sciences. 2025;**16**(Suppl 5):S4572–S4574. DOI: 10.4103/jpbs.jpbs_927_24

[12] Daneshjou R, Vodrahalli K, Novoa RA, Jenkins M, Liang W, Rotemberg V, Justin K, Swetter SM, Bailey EE, Gevaert O, Mukherjee P, Phung M, Yekrang K, Fong B, Sahasrabudhe R, Allerup JAC, Okata-Karigane U, Zou J, Chiou AS. Disparities in dermatology AI performance on a diverse, curated clinical image set. Science Advances. 2022;**8**(32):eabq6147. DOI: 10.1126/sciadv.abq6147

[13] Char DS, Shah NH, Magnus D. Implementing machine learning in health care—addressing ethical challenges. New England Journal of Medicine. 2018;**378**(11):981–983

[14] Kavouras I, Gomez T, Chalbot MC. UVA and cutaneous melanoma

incidences: Spatial patterns and communities at risk. Journal of Environmental Health. 2015;**77**(9):8–14

[15] Elder DE, Massi D, Scolyer RA, Willemze R. WHO Classification of Skin Tumours. Lyon: IARC; 2018

[16] Marghoob AA, Braun RP. Atlas of Dermoscopy. 2nd ed. Boca Raton (FL): CRC Press; 2011

[17] Ciudad-Blancoa C, Avilés-Izquierdoa JA, Lázaro-Ochaitab P, Suárez-Fernándeza R. Dermoscopic findings for the early detection of melanoma: An analysis of 200 cases. Actas Dermo-Sifiliográficas. 2014;**105**:635–8. DOI: 10.1016/j.adengl.2014.07.015

[18] Voloshynovych M, Pietkiewicz P, Navarette-Dechent C, Lallas A, Paoli J, Kittler H, Marghoob AA, Goldust M, Szepietowski JC, Zalaudek I, Beachkofsky TM, Longo C, Rosendahl C, Kiss N, Argenziano G, Jafferany M, Leszczyńska-Pietkiewicz A, Salwowska N, Matkovska N. Dermoscopic image digital post-processing perception and use among members of the international dermoscopy society: Results of a web-based survey. Dermatology Practical & Conceptual. 2025;**15**(3):5366. DOI: 10.5826/dpc.1503a5366

[19] Pizzichetta MA, Talamini R, Piccolo D, et al. Amelanotic/hypomelanotic melanoma: Clinical and dermoscopic features. British Journal of Dermatology. 2004;**150**:1117–1124

[20] Thomas NE, Kricker A, Waxweiler WT, et al. Comparison of clinicopathologic features and survival of histopathologically amelanotic and pigmented melanomas. JAMA Dermatology. 2014;**150**:1306–1314

[21] Dessinioti C, Antoniou C, Katsambas A, Stratigos AJ.Basal cell carcinoma: What's new under the sun. Photochemistry and Photobiology. 2010;**86**(3):481–491

[22] Hafner C, Vogt T. Seborrheic keratosis. JDDG: Journal der Deutschen Dermatologischen Gesellschaft. 2008;**6**(8):664–677

[23] Carrera C, Segura S, Aguilera P, et al. Dermoscopic clues for diagnosing melanomas that resemble seborrheic keratosis. JAMA Dermatology. 2017;**153**:544–551

[24] Minagawa A. Dermoscopy-pathology relationship in seborrheic keratosis. Journal of Dermatology. 2017;**44**(5):518–524. DOI: 10.1111/1346-8138.13657

[25] Michalak-Stoma A, Małkińska K, Krasowska D. Usefulness of dermoscopy to provide accurate assessment of skin cancers. Clinical, Cosmetic and Investigational Dermatology. 2021;**14**:733–746. DOI: 10.2147/CCID.S305924

[26] Lallas A, Apalla Z, Argenziano G, et al. The dermatoscopic universe of basal cell carcinoma. Dermatology Practical & Conceptual. 2014;**4**:11–24

[27] Wollina U. Recent advances in managing and understanding seborrheic keratosis. F1000Research. 2019;**8**:1520

[28] Forsea AM.Melanoma epidemiology and early detection in Europe: Diversity and disparities. Dermatology Practical & Conceptual. 2020;**10**(3):e2020033

[29] Forsea AM, Del Marmol V, Stratigos A, Geller AC. Melanoma

prognosis in Europe: Far from equal. British Journal of Dermatology. 2014;**171**(1):179–182

[30] Gupta AK, Bharadwaj M, Mehrotra R. Skin cancer concerns in people of color: Risk factors and diagnostic challenges. Dermatologic Clinics. 2022;**40**(3):313–321

[31] Agbai ON, Buster K, Sanchez M, et al. Skin cancer and photoprotection in people of color: A review and recommendations for physicians and the public. Journal of the American Academy of Dermatology. 2014;**70**: 748–762

[32] Tschandl P, Codella N, Akay BN, et al. Comparison of the accuracy of human readers versus machine-learning algorithms for pigmented skin lesion classification: An open, web-based, international, diagnostic study. The Lancet Oncology. 2019;**20**:938–947

[33] Esteva A, Robicquet A, Ramsundar B, et al. A guide to deep learning in healthcare. Nature Medicine. 2019;**25**:24–29

[34] Brinker TJ, Hekler A, Enk AH, et al. Deep learning outperformed 136 of 157 dermatologists in a head-to-head dermoscopic melanoma image classification task. European Journal of Cancer. 2019;**113**:47–54

[35] Tan M, Le Q. EfficientNet: Rethinking model scaling for convolutional neural networks. Proceedings of Machine Learning Research. 2019;**97**:6105–6114

[36] Aswath R, Pankaj S, Vasant PV. Role of dermoscopy in diagnosing and differentiating seborrheic keratoses a case study of 100 patients. Egyptian Journal of Dermatology and Venerology. 2022;**42**(3):174–182. DOI: 10.4103/ejdv.ejdv_39_21

[37] Celebi ME, Kingravi HA, Iyatomi H, Aslandogan YA, Stoecker WV, Moss RH, et al. A methodological approach to the classification of dermoscopy images. Computerized Medical Imaging and Graphics. 2007;**31**:362–373

[38] Haenssle HA, Fink C, Schneiderbauer R, Toberer F, Buhl T, Enk A, Kalloo A, Hassen ABH, Thomas L, Enk A, et al. Melanoma recognition by a deep learning convolutional neural network—Performance in different melanoma subtypes and localisations. European Journal of Cancer. 2020;**127**:21–29

[39] Lu C, Mahmood T.Deep learning applications in pathology. Nature Reviews Clinical Oncology. 2020;**17** (12):703–715

[40] Viknesh CK, Kumar PN, Seetharaman R, Anitha D. Detection and classification of melanoma skin cancer using image processing technique. Diagnostics (Basel). 2023;**13** (21):3313. DOI: 10.3390/diagnostics13213313

[41] Frid-Adar M, Klang E, Amitai M, Goldberger J, Greenspan H. Synthetic data augmentation using GAN for improved liver lesion classification. IEEE Transactions on Medical Imaging. 2018;**38**(3):677–685

[42] Han SS, Kim MS, Lim W, GH P, Park I, Chang SE. Classification of the clinical images for benign and malignant cutaneous tumors using a deep learning algorithm. Journal of Investigative Dermatology. 2018;**138**(7):1529–1538

[43] Islam S, Wishart GC, Walls J, Hall P, Seco de Herrera AG, Gan JQ, Raza H. Advancing skin cancer detection through deep learning and fusion of patient metadata and skin lesion images. Scientific Reports. 2026;**16**:1968. DOI: 10.1038/s41598-025-26392-4

[44] Combalia M, Codella N, Rotemberg V, et al. BCN20000: Dermoscopic Lesions in the Wild. arXiv Preprint. 2019

[45] Bissoto A, Fornaciali M, Valle E, Avila S. (De)constructing bias on skin lesion datasets. Conference on Computer Vision and Pattern Recognition Workshops. IEEE Computer Society Conference on Computer Vision and Pattern Recognition. Workshops. 2019

[46] Berry E, Thompson RF, Shachaf C, Leachman S. Molecular imaging in early skin cancer detection: Advances, limitations, and future directions. Technology in Cancer Research & Treatment. 2025;**24**:15330338251410073. DOI: 10.1177/15330338251410073

[47] Haenssle HA, Fink C, Schneiderbauer R, et al. Man against machine: Diagnostic performance of a deep learning convolutional neural network for dermoscopic melanoma recognition. Annals of Oncology. 2018;**29**:1836–1842

[48] Marchetti MA, Codella NC, Dusza SW, et al. Results of the 2016 International Skin Imaging Collaboration International Symposium on Biomedical Imaging challenge. JAMA Dermatology. 2017;**153**:1282–1286

[49] Adamson AS, Smith A.Machine learning and health care disparities in dermatology. JAMA Dermatology. 2018;**154**(11):1247–1248

[50] Liu Y, Jain A, Eng C, et al. A deep learning system for differential diagnosis of skin diseases. Nature Medicine. 2020;**26**:900–908

[51] Cancer Genome Atlas Network. Genomic classification of cutaneous melanoma. Cell. 2015;**161**(7): 1681–1696

[52] Roufas C, Georgakopoulos-Soares I, Zaravinos A. Distinct genomic features across cytolytic subgroups in skin melanoma. Cancer Immunology, Immunotherapy. 2021;**70**:3137–3154. DOI: 10.1007/s00262-021-02918-3

[53] Brinker TJ, Hekler A, Hauschild A, et al. Comparing artificial intelligence algorithms to 157 German dermatologists: The melanoma classification benchmark. European Journal of Cancer. 2019;**111**:30–37

[54] Freeman K, Dinnes J, Chuchu N, et al. Algorithm-based smartphone apps to assess risk of skin cancer in adults: Systematic review of diagnostic accuracy studies. BMJ. 2020;**368**:m127

[55] Venkatesh KP, Kadakia KT, Gilbert S. Learnings from the first AI-enabled skin cancer device for primary care authorized by FDA. NPJ Digital Medicine. 2024;**7**:156. DOI: 10.1038/s41746-024-01161-1

[56] Cui M, Zhang DY. Artificial intelligence and computational pathology. Laboratory Investigation. 2021;**101**(4):412–422

[57] Lui H, Zhao J, McLean D, Zeng H. Real-time raman spectroscopy for

in vivo skin cancer diagnosis. Cancer Research. 2012;**72**(10):2491–2500

[58] Madarkar SS, Madarkar M, Madhumitha V, et al. DermaCon-IN: A Multi-concept Annotated Dermatological Image Dataset of Indian Skin Disorders for Clinical AI Research. Available from: https://arxiv.org/abs/2506.06099 [Accessed: 2025-July-20]

[59] Vossaert K, Lanssens S, Beirens A, Van Vaerenbergh N, Coussens E. The TRIAGE and ASSIST scan: A new concept in 3D total body imaging for early melanoma detection. European Journal of Cancer – Skin Cancer Section. 2025;**3**:100748. DOI: 10.1016/j.ejcskn.2025.100748

[60] Ongena YP, Haan M, Yakar D, Kwee TC. Patients' views on the implementation of artificial intelligence in radiology: Development and validation of a standardized questionnaire. European Radiology. 2020;**30**(2):1033–1040

[61] Vellido A. Societal issues concerning the application of artificial intelligence in medicine. Kidney Diseases. 2019;**5**(1):11–17

[62] Pacheco AGC, Krohling RA. The impact of patient clinical information on automated skin cancer detection. Computers in Biology and Medicine. 2020;**116**:103545. DOI: 10.1016/j.compbiomed.2019.103545

[63] Rudin C. Stop explaining black box models for high stakes decisions and use interpretable models instead. Nature Machine Intelligence. 2019;**1**(5):206–215

[64] Lepère P, Tchounga B, Ekouevi D-K. Digital health in francophone Sub-Saharan Africa: Catching up! Médecine Et Santé Tropicales. 2017;**27**(4):342–345. DOI: 10.1684/mst.2017.0724

[65] Al-Waisy AS, Al-Fahdawi S, Khalaf MI, Mohammed MA, Al-Attar B, Al-Andoli MN. A deep learning framework for automated early diagnosis and classification of skin cancer lesions in dermoscopy images. Scientific Reports. 2025;**15**:31234. DOI: 10.1038/s41598-025-15655-9

[66] Chanda T, Haggenmueller S, Bucher T-C, Holland-Letz T, Kittler H, Tschandl P, Heppt MV, Berking C, Utikal JS, Schilling B, Buerger C, Navarrete-Dechent C, Goebeler M, Kather JN, Schneider CV, Durani B, Durani H, Jansen M, Wacker J, Wacker J, Consortium RS, Brinker TJ. Dermatologist-like explainable AI enhances melanoma diagnosis accuracy: Eye-tracking study. Nature Communications. 2025;**16**:4739. DOI: 10.1038/s41467-025-59532-5

[67] Topol EJ. High-performance medicine: The convergence of human and artificial intelligence. Nature Medicine. 2019;**25**(1):44–56

[68] Cukras AR. On the comparison of diagnosis and management of melanoma between dermatologists and MelaFind. JAMADermatol. 2013;**149**:622–623

[69] Ollmar S, Grant S. Nevisense: Improving the accuracy of diagnosing melanoma. Melanoma Management. 2016;**3**:93–96

[70] Wang XM, Borsky K, Proctor DW, Goodall R, Marshall DC, Dobell W, Salciccioli JD, Matin RN, Shalhoub J, El-Muttardi N. Trends in cutaneous melanoma mortality and incidence in

European Union 15+ countries between 1990 and 2019. Journal of the European Academy of Dermatology and Venereology (JEADV). 2025;**39**(7):1285-1296. DOI: 10.1111/jdv.20524

[71] Heinlein L, Maron RC, Hekler A, Haggenmüller S, Wies C, Utikal JS, Meier F, Hobelsberger S, Gellrich FF, Sergon M, Hauschild A, French LE, Heinzerling L, Schlager JG, Ghoreschi K, Schlaak M, Hilke FJ, Poch G, Korsing S, Berking C, Heppt MV, Erdmann M, Haferkamp S, Drexler K, Schadendorf D, Sondermann W, Goebeler M, Schilling B, Krieghoff-Henning E, Brinker TJ. Prospective multicenter study using artificial intelligence to improve dermoscopic melanoma diagnosis in patient care. Communication Medicine. 2024;**4**:177. DOI: 10.1038/s43856-024-00598-5